FOOD SCIENCE AND TECHNOLOGY

FUNCTIONAL FOODS

SOURCES, BIOTECHNOLOGY APPLICATIONS AND HEALTH CHALLENGES

FOOD SCIENCE AND TECHNOLOGY

Additional books in this series can be found on Nova's website
under the Series tab.

Additional e-books in this series can be found on Nova's website
under the e-book tab.

NUTRITION AND DIET RESEARCH PROGRESS

Additional books in this series can be found on Nova's website
under the Series tab.

Additional e-books in this series can be found on Nova's website
under the e-book tab.

FOOD SCIENCE AND TECHNOLOGY

FUNCTIONAL FOODS

SOURCES, BIOTECHNOLOGY APPLICATIONS AND HEALTH CHALLENGES

ARON ROBINSON
AND
DOMINICK EMERSON
EDITORS

nova publishers
New York

For permission to use material from this book please contact us:
Telephone 631-231-7269; Fax 631-231-8175
Web Site: http://www.novapublishers.com

Library of Congress Cataloging-in-Publication Data

Functional foods : sources, biotechnology applications, and health challenges / [edited by] Aron Robinson and Dominick Emerson.
pages cm
Includes bibliographical references and index.
ISBN: 978-1-62417-435-3 (hardcover)
1. Functional foods. 2. Food--Biotechnology. 3. Nutrition. I. Robinson, Aron, editor of compilation. II. Emerson, Dominick, editor of compilation.
QP144.F85F859 2013
613.2--dc23

2012044112

Published by Nova Science Publishers, Inc. † New York

CONTENTS

PREFACE

In this book, the authors discuss the sources, biotechnology applications and health challenges of functional foods. Topics discussed include the health potential of pulses and their bioactivity; health promoting phytonutrients and lactic acid bacteria in olives; health benefits of the Mediterranean diet; European consumers acceptance of healthy food products; fermentation of tomato juice with the probiotic yeast saccharomyces cerevisiae boulardii; and market strategies to maximize consumer acceptance of functional dairy-based foods and beverages.

Chapter 1 – The maintenance of health and the prevention and treatment of chronic diseases are influenced by naturally occurring chemicals in foods. In addition to supplying the substrates for producing energy, many dietary chemicals are bioactive; they alter the regulation of biological processes and expression of genetic information. Pulses are legume seeds used for human consumption and include peas, beans, lentils, chickpeas, and faba beans. In addition to being a source of macronutrients and minerals, pulses also contain plant secondary metabolites that are increasingly being recognized for their potential benefits for human health. Emerging evidence stresses the importance of pulses as carriers of several constituents of potential biological importance, including enzyme inhibitors, lectins, phytates, oxalates, polyphenols, saponins and phytosterols.

Recent investigations suggest that pulses may contribute to human health and wellbeing, mostly through prevention of chronic diseases such as coronary heart disease, hypertension, cancer, diabetes and obesity. The mechanisms responsible for this apparently protective role may include gene-nutrient interactions. Taking advantage of the above, great efforts have recently been invested to potentiate their technological use on the development of healthful ingredients, such as flour mixtures and extruded snacks, aimed to create functional and healthy food. This chapter investigates the health potential of pulses, examining their bioactivity, highlighting the studies involving functional compounds that modulate genes for prevention of diseases as well as their potential use in industry.

Chapter 2 – Available scientific evidence supports claims issued on a few foods (or food components) about their favourable role upon human health – beyond merely responding to basic nutritional requirements. A stronger and stronger consumer awareness has meanwhile shifted to such a tertiary role of foods, especially in view of their efficacy to specifically address chronic diseases and health conditions – including ageing.

Some foods marketed as functional are actually natural whole foods (e.g. plant-based foods, such as fruits, vegetables and whole grains) containing significant amounts of bioactive phytochemicals for which new scientific information was released focusing on their effects upon health; in many instances, functionality of already existing foods needs only be publicized at large. In particular, the fruits of the olive tree (Olea europaea L.) have been for ages consumed as such, or else used as feedstock for oil production; although such a consumption stems solely from nutritional features as part of a regular Mediterranean diet, it has been reported that olive fruits contain 1–3% of their fresh pulp weight of insoluble, or water- and lipid-soluble compounds bearing multiple biological properties – e.g. antioxidant, anticarcinogenic, anti-inflammatory, antimicrobial, antihypertensive, antilipidemic, cardiotonic, laxative and anti-platelet aggregation.

Furthermore, table olives may be considered as effective carriers (and even as a wild source) of lactic acid bacteria bearing probiotic features. Such adventitious strains belong to the Lactobacillus genus – and exhibit a remarkable capacity to tolerate the high acidity and salt content of fermented vegetables, as well as an ability to adhere to the colon wall and survive transit through the gastrointestinal tract. This realization may lead to improvements in the technological aspects of fermentative processing, and as well as emphasize the inherent functional value of fermented table olives – i.e. combine food safety and proactive contribution to human health in a novel manner.

Therefore, this chapter addresses a novel probiotic food by comprehensively and critically reviewing available information on health-promoting phytonutrients and lactic acid bacteria in olives, aiming at a better understanding of its potential toward improvement of health – thus consubstantiating a case study of a plant-based functional food.

Chapter 3 – The Mediterranean diet is a well recognized life and food habits having relevant association with a reduced mortality caused by diseases such as cardiovascular disease, obesity, diabetes, cancer and neurodegenerative disorders. The importance of a healthy balanced diet lies on the fact that benefits come from the presence and the interaction of almost all the nutrients with which it is composed. It is a matter of fact that single nutrients can behave differently from what it is observed when they are all mixed together with interactive possibility. Under this perspective, the Mediterranean diet is both composed by a great number of single functional food and, as a whole, it is a result of a balance between the single nutrient properties, as evidenced by its great capacity to prevent all the chronic degenerative disorders above mentioned. Among the functional food present in the Mediterranean diet are cereals, legumes, fruit and vegetables, nuts, olive oil as the prevalent fats for dressing, red wine in moderate quantity and consumed at meals, fish and poultry as the main source of protein and polyunsaturated/saturated fats, modest quantity of dairy products, spices. Since the Mediterranean diet is a dietary pattern common to more than one country in the Mediterranean basin, some differences can be found between the food consumed by the populations. The health benefits coming from the food of the Mediterranean diet resides on the presence of bioactive compounds such as polyphenols, carotenoids, phytosterols, fibers, monounsaturated and polyunsaturated fatty acids, displaying antioxidant activity, protection from cancer and hypertension, improvement of the immune response. Due to the presence of more than one functional food groups in the same dietary pattern, sometimes in the same meal, diverse species of polyphenols as well as of phytosterols, fibers and fatty acids can be combined and activated. Next to the positive properties derived from the food, the physical activity also account for an important aspect of this life habits. In fact, since lifestyle modification programs provide a method to change eating and activity habits, any diet intervention becomes more valid with a regular daily physical activity.

The last element characterizing the Mediterranean diet is the perception of a meal as a moment to spend with other people and of food as a positive link. For all these complex and heterogeneous aspects, the Mediterranean diet has recently been named as "intangible cultural heritage by UNESCO".

Chapter 4 – In the recent past, Europe has experienced an increase in several chronic diseases linked to dietary and lifestyle habits. In particular, obesity is continuously increasing at an alarming rate all over Europe. As a result healthier food products have rapidly gained important market shares. The food industry has rapidly reacted to this trend by developing a growing variety of new products with health-related claims and images, including functional foods (FF) that are selected by consumers for their health-promoting properties. However, demand for FF within the European Union varies considerably from country to country, mainly due to food traditions and different cultural heritage. This chapter offers an overview of the current FF market situation in Europe and addresses the main cognitive, motivational and attitudinal determinants of consumer acceptance of these foods in different European countries, providing practical insights of the profile of FF consumers. In particular, the major factors that are currently restraining growth of FF in Europe (beyond economic crisis) are highlighted and deeply discussed. As the lack of categorisation (it is still difficult for consumers to distinguish between functional and conventional food products); growing consumer confusion (due to increasing product variety and product labelling, together with the overwhelming amount of general marketing and educational messages on food intake); low awareness of health benefits of functional ingredients; lack of consensus on the level of scientific support and documentation required for specific health claims. The current work could help practitioners in making more effective strategic and tactical marketing decisions, and add some useful information for government bodies interested in designing public health programs.

Chapter 5 – A new functional beverage based on tomato juice fermented with the probiotic yeast *Saccharomyces cerevisiae boulardii* was formulated. Viability of the yeast, assayed after 24 h of incubation in the tomato juice and over 56 days of storage of the fermented product at 4°C, was comparable to that obtained by culturing the yeast in potato dextrose broth, used as a control. Therefore, the different culturing media did not negatively affect the yeast resistance to the *in vitro* passage through acidic and pancreatic environment. Some biochemical parameters of the fermented juice, polyphenol and lycopene content, as well as its DPPH free radical scavenging capability, were evaluated during storage and under *in vitro*-simulated gastrointestinal conditions. Fermentation of the juice with *S. boulardii* caused only a slight decrease of total polyphenols (0.442 μmol/μl *versus* 0.474 μmol/μl, respectively) and lycopene (13.38 μg/ml *versus* 16.76 μg/ml, respectively), compared to the raw juice. On the other hand, after passage through *in vitro* double gastric+ pancreatic conditions, the amount of such bio-components was constant during storage until 28 days, decreasing only after 56 days. Probably, such behaviour affected the slight loss of DPPH radical scavenging activity of the fermented juice with respect to the fresh product, and a decrease of 14% with respect to the initial value (EC_{50}= 38.54 μl) was observed after 56 days of storage (EC_{50}= 44.36 μl), although, after the double *in vitro* gastric+pancreatic passage, the amount of fermented juice request to inhibit the DPPH activity of 50% increased three times. The developed product might represent another example of an alternative for delivering probiotics, especially for individuals suffering from lactose intolerance to dairy products.

Chapter 6 – The food industry generally, and the dairy industry specifically, are for the most part low-margin and extremely competitive businesses. Recent dairy industry trends have centered on food safety, product differentiation through quality, rigorous cost containment, careful inventory management, innovation management, and channel complexity (including the growing influence of retailers on the supply chain). However, as the demand for commodity dairy decreases in Western Europe, demand for dairy that offers health benefits - functional dairy - has never been greater. Dairy products can have vastly different characteristics, ranging from beverage to powder, solid to viscous, canned, bagged and boxed. Ingredients found in these products have been associated with a wide variety of health benefits and have been incorporated into a number of non-dairy based food and beverages as a means of increasing overall nutritional profile of the product. Consumer's increasing interest for maintaining and/or improving their health by eating these specific food products has led to the development of many new functional dairy products. However, not all of these products are met with consumer acceptance and product failure rate remains high. As sales of commodity dairy products slow in Western Europe, strategies that maximise and increase consumer acceptance of functional dairy foods and dairy ingredients are necessary to ensure a sustainable competitive advantage and ensure growth.

In: Functional Foods
Editors: Aron Robinson and Dominick Emerson
ISBN: 978-1-62417-435-3

Chapter 1

PULSES FACING THE NEW AGE: FUNCTIONAL COMPOUNDS ON GENE EXPRESSION AND HEALTH CONNECTION

Hayde Azeneth Vergara-Castañeda[1], B. Dave Oomah[2] and Rocio Campos-Vega[1,3,*]

[1]Programa de Posgrado en Alimentos del Centro de la República (PROPAC), Research and Graduate Studies in Food Science, School of Chemistry, Universidad Autónoma de Querétaro, Querétaro, Qro, México

[2]National Bioproducts and Bioprocesses Program, Pacific Agri-Food Research Centre, Agriculture and Agri-Food Canada, Summerland, British Columbia, Canada

[3]Kellogg de México, Carretera al Campo Militar, San Antonio de la Punta, Querétaro, Qro., México

ABSTRACT

The maintenance of health and the prevention and treatment of chronic diseases are influenced by naturally occurring chemicals in foods. In addition to supplying the substrates for producing energy, many dietary chemicals are bioactive; they alter the regulation of biological processes and expression of genetic information. Pulses are legume seeds used for human consumption and include peas, beans, lentils, chickpeas, and faba beans. In addition to being a source of macronutrients and minerals, pulses also contain plant secondary metabolites that are increasingly being recognized for their potential benefits for human health. Emerging evidence stresses the importance of pulses as carriers of several constituents of potential biological importance, including enzyme inhibitors, lectins, phytates, oxalates, polyphenols, saponins and phytosterols.

Recent investigations suggest that pulses may contribute to human health and wellbeing, mostly through prevention of chronic diseases such as coronary heart disease, hypertension, cancer, diabetes and obesity. The mechanisms responsible for this apparently protective role may include gene-nutrient interactions. Taking advantage of

* Corresponding author: telephone (442) 211 1400 Ext 1720. *E-mail address*: rocio.campos@kellogg.com; chio_cve@yahoo.com.mx.

the above, great efforts have recently been invested to potentiate their technological use on the development of healthful ingredients, such as flour mixtures and extruded snacks, aimed to create functional and healthy food. This chapter investigates the health potential of pulses, examining their bioactivity, highlighting the studies involving functional compounds that modulate genes for prevention of diseases as well as their potential use in industry.

INTRODUCTION

Pulses are regarded as a beneficial source of nutrients and are recommended as a staple food by health organizations and dieticians. They are rich sources of vitamins, minerals and carbohydrates in the human diet. Pulses represent an important source of protein for vegetarians, are low glycemic index food and also recognized as food choice with significant potential health benefits. They are excellent foods for people managing their diabetes, heart disease or celiac disease, and additionally can help people concerned with weight control. Moreover, the interest in the utilization of pulses in the developed world is on the increase. In an effort to improve the nutrition of many developing countries, or to combat the incidence of various chronic diseases worldwide, food technologists have developed products based on pulses, adding value thereby contributing to increase in the consumption of legumes. This chapter provides a comprehensive assessment of the nutrition and health aspects of pulses, and describes many current technological applications that have been developed based on legumes.

BEANS

Common bean (*Phaseolus vulgaris* L.) is a seed widely distributed around the world and mainly in Latin America and Africa. Common bean is rich in proteins, carbohydrates, dietary fiber (soluble and insoluble) and low in fat, that is rich in linoleic acid. Beans are considered a good source of vitamins (thiamine, riboflavin, niacin, vitamin B_6 and folic acid) and some minerals (calcium, magnesium, iron, phosphorus, potassium and zinc) (Serrano and Goñi, 2004). Consumption of common beans contributes to the prevention and/or treatment of degenerative-chronic diseases, such as obesity, diabetes, cancer, cardiovascular diseases, partly due to the influence of micronutrients (mainly folic acid and magnesium) and high fiber content, condensed tannins, phytoestrogens and non-essential amino acids (Rodríguez-Castillo and Fernández-Rojas, 2003).

Common beans are a good source of aromatic amino acids, lysine, leucine and isoleucine, but deficient in sulfur amino acids (methionine and cysteine), valine, tryptophan and threonine. However, beans are usually consumed with corn tortilla, which is a good complementation of both proteins, resulting in a protein with high nutritional value (Serrano and Goñi, 2004). Components of common beans considered non-nutritive are enzyme inhibitors (trypsin and α-amylase), phytates, oxalates, phenolic compounds, saponins, and others. However, it has been shown that all these compounds may have beneficial effects on health; for this reason several authors have classified them as bioactive compounds in common beans (Jenab and Thompson, 2002; Kennedy et al., 2002; Serrano and Goñi, 2004, Gálvez-Ranilla et al., 2007; Oboh and Omofomà, 2008).

Nutraceutical Properties of Beans

Common bean consumption as a fiber source increase satiety due to increased food volume, long intestinal transit time, which produces more sensation of intestinal fullness; high levels of cholecystokinin hormone, related to reduced glucose and insulin levels in plasma of diabetic patients (Bourdon et al., 2001). Moreover, bean intake also has hypocholesterolemic effect because of its fiber content, which influences lipoproteins level by decreasing low density lipoproteins. Bazzano et al., (2001) found a strong inverse relationship between legume intake and risk of coronary heart disease (CHD); and soluble fiber is considered the major component responsible for this benefit, as well as better glycemic control (Rimm et al., 1996). Beans are a major source of dietary folate (Messina, 1999). Both folate and vitamin B12 are important for homocysteine metabolism, and dietary intake of folate has been inversely associated with plasma homocysteine levels (Selhub et al., 1993), which at elevated levels is related to increased risk of CHD.

Bean consumption has also been associated with alteration of bile acids and sterols excretion, fat digestibility coefficient reduction (Duane, 1997), as well as increase in the production of short chain fatty acids during colonic fermentation (Sengupta et al., 2006). Dietary components that are not digested in the upper intestinal tract and endogenous glycans (mucins, glycosphingolipids) are the main nutrients for microflora living in the distal small intestine and colon. Among these, the complex carbohydrate (oligo-and poly-saccharides) supplied by the diet are the most abundant group of substrates fermentable by the flora (Sanz et al., 2004). These carbohydrates are hydrolyzed and fermented by intestinal bacteria, producing gases and mostly short-chain fatty acids such as acetic, propionic and butyric acids (Granito et al., 2001). Campos-Vega et al., (2009) reported the fiber content ranging from 36.5% to 55% in cooked Negro 8025, Bayo Madero, Pinto Durango and Azufrado Higuera beans grown in Mexico, , while the range in raw beans was 25.6-37.6%. The soluble fiber content ranged from 5.5-14% and 0.3-1.6%, whereas the insoluble fiber content was 31-41% and 25.2-36.1% in cooked and raw beans, respectively. Soluble fiber mixed with water produces a lattice which is trapped, resulting in solutions with high viscosity. This viscosity acts on lipid metabolism with anticarcinogenic effects. Insoluble fiber retains water in its structural matrix forming mixtures of low viscosity, increasing faecal mass, speeding intestinal transit and decreasing the concentration and contact time of carcinogens with the colon mucosa (Escudero-Álvarez and González-Sánchez, 2006).

Dietary fiber, specifically the soluble fraction, reduces serum cholesterol and LDL concentrations, which may contribute to its protective role against heart disease (Anderson et al., 1995). Thus, one serving per day of beans has been associated with a 38% lower risk of myocardial infarction (Kabagambe et al., 2005). Furthermore, individuals consuming legumes at least 4 times per week can lower their risk of heart disease by 22% than those consuming legumes less than once per week (Bazzano et al., 2001). Anderson et al., (1984) fed hyperlipidemic men 120–162 g/d pinto beans and reported that bean diets decreased serum cholesterol concentrations by 19% and low-density lipoprotein cholesterol by 24%, concluding that bean supplements may have an important role in nutritional management of selected hypercholesterolemic patients. In another study, Fruhbeck et al., (1997) examined the hypocholesterolemic effect and hormonal changes resulting from 90 g/d supplementation with *Vicia faba* L. (field bean) flour in the diets of young men for 30 d. Field bean supplementation significantly reduced serum glucose, insulin, triacylglycerol, total-, LDL- and very-low-density-lipoprotein (VLDL)-cholesterol values in all subjects and increased glucagon and high-density-lipoprotein cholesterol levels. Krupa-Kozak et al., (2010) tested a bean starch isolated from bean seeds (*Phaseolus vulgaris*) cultivar Laponia on serum biochemical markers in rats. Bean starch significantly reduced the total cholesterol concentration without lowering the HDL-cholesterol fraction and there was a considerable reduction in glucose. Kintoni bean (*Phaseolus vulgaris*) elevated fecal bile acid excretions and reduced the serum total cholesterol, HDL-cholesterol, and VLDL + IDL + LDL-cholesterol concentrations by fecal steroid excretion accelerated by *n*-butyrate and increased hepatic LDL receptor, SR-B1, and cholesterol 7α-hydroxylase mRNAs (Figure 1) (Han et al., 2004). Adzuki bean resistant starch has a serum cholesterol-lowering function via enhancement of the hepatic LDL-receptor mRNA, cholesterol 7α-hydroxylase mRNA levels and faecal bile acid excretion, and decrease in the hepatic HMG-CoA reductase mRNA level in rats when added to a cholesterol diet (Han et al., 2006).

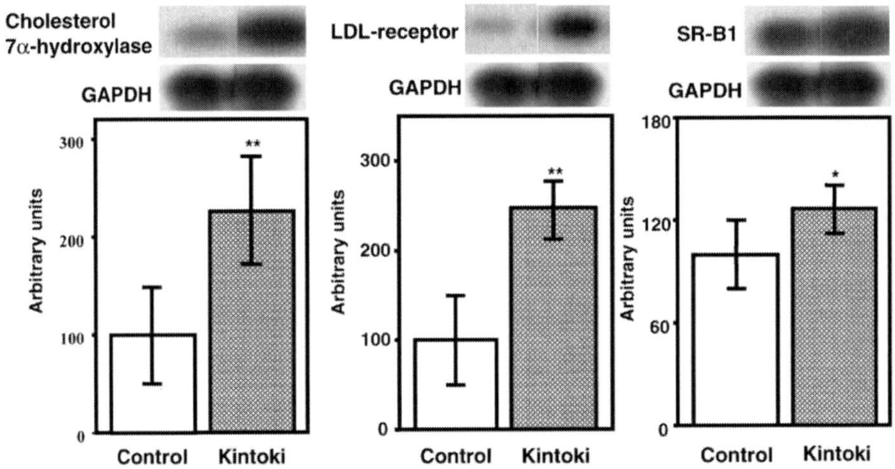

Figure 1. Hepatic cholesterol 7α-hydroxylase mRNA, LDL receptor mRNA, and SR-B1 mRNA levels in rats fed pancreatin-resistant fraction prepared from kintoki bean for 4 weeks. Values are means for five rats, with standard deviations indicated by bars. *P <0.05, **P<0.01 versus control. Control, cellulose powder; kintoki, pancreatin-resistant fraction prepared from kintoki bean (Adapted from Han et al., 2004).

Furthermore, because of the low glycaemic index (GI) and the high content of undigestible fibres, dry beans are claimed to help glycaemic control in diabetic individuals. Dry legumes may prevent insulin-resistance, which represents the presyndrome to type II diabetes (Duranti, 2006). Beans are the perfect food to improve glycemic control with low glycemic index, varying from 27-42% relative to glucose and 40-59% that of white bread. Substituting beans for foods prepared from white flour (on an equal dry weight basis) will reduce the glycemic index of the diet by about two-thirds and glycemic load by about 80%. Furthermore, consuming beans will significantly increase intake of dietary fiber that is particularly important for controlling blood glucose concentrations (Foster-Powell and Miller,

1995). In type 2 diabetic subjects, ingestion of kidney beans resulted in a significantly lower glucose area compared to ingestion of 50 g glucose (Krezowski et al., 1987). In experimental animals, the administration of blackgram fiber (30% neutral detergent fiber) diet showed a significant increase in liver glycogen level and reduced hepatic gluconeogenesis (Jenkins et al., 2002). The consumption of a diet containing raw kidney beans significantly affects the amount of insulin receptor and GLUT-4 mRNAs present in skeletal muscle in rats, where the increase in GLUT-4 mRNA and insulin receptor mRNA levels may play a role in the modulatory process (Knott et al., 1992). Dry beans are also rich in phytates, soluble fiber and tannins, all of which correlate inversely with carbohydrate digestion and glycemic response (Liener, 1994).

Experimental data indicates the beneficial effects of both fiber fractions (indigestible carbohydrates) on the reduction of cancer incidence in animal models such as *in vitro* experiments. The protection afforded by this compound is through inhibition of carcinogens activation, prevention of mutations, and apoptotic activation (Niba and Niba, 2003). Hangen and Bennink (2002) showed that black and navy beans consumption significantly reduces colon cancer incidence and tumor multiplicity in azoxymethane (AOM)-induced rats. A prospective cohort study found that eating beans and lentils significantly reduced the risk of prostate cancer (Mills et al., 1989). Krupa-Kozak et al., (2010) showed that adding bean starch preparations to diets increased the amount of N excreted in faeces, with a simultaneous decrease in the coefficient of apparent N digestibility, which probably indicates increased bacteria proliferation of *Bifidobacterium spp.* and *Lactobacillus spp.* in the large intestine. There were also an increased concentration and pool of SCFA including acetic, propionic and butyric acids in the caecum of rats fed diets with bean starch preparations, as well as reduced activity of potentially harmful β-glucuronidase. Such an effect should be considered as beneficial because β-glucuronidase has the ability to hydrolyze many glucuronide conjugates and thus may release active carcinogenic metabolites in the intestinal lumen (Rafter, 2002). Vergara-Castañeda et al., (2010) also demonstrated that common bean (cv. Bayo Madero) and its non-digestible fraction reduced β-glucuronidase activity in AOM-induced rats, thereby indicating a strong probiotic effect exerted by these compounds. Moreover, the scientific community has attempted to elucidate the molecular pathways involved in the beneficial effects to attack cancer at different stages of the disease. Feregrino-Pérez et al., (2008) reported that the polysaccharides extract from common beans Negro 8025 cultivar contains considerable amounts of non-digested carbohydrates (mostly soluble and insoluble fiber) that are fermented in the large intestine producing SCFA, mainly butyrate, resulting in a decrease in aberrant crypt foci development in distal colon of AOM-induced rats. The authors suggested that such lesion development was prevented by the modulation of the expression of genes involved in proliferation, cellular arrest, and apoptosis (β-catenin, p53, p21, Rb, Bax, and Caspase-3).

Thompson et al., (2012) demonstrated that a high common bean (60% wt/wt) diet , may decrease the carcinoma burden in bean-fed rats by 62.2% due most predominantly to induction of apoptosis based on histological and western blot analyses. Anti-apoptotic factors Bcl-2 and X-linked inhibitor of apoptosis protein decreased in mammary carcinomas of bean-fed rats; whereas pro-apoptotic factors Bax and apoptosis protease-activating factor-1 increased with bean consumption. In addition, the authors found a modification in key metabolic signaling networks linked to cell growth and survival. Adenosine monophosphate-activated protein kinase (AMPK) was activated and acetyl-CoA carboxylase (ACC) was downregulated. The AMPK-mediated suppression of ACC activity limits the ability of the cell to carry out robust lipid synthesis required for tumor growth. The protective effect of common beans against cancer has also been demonstrated on *in vitro* models, using several cell lines. For instance, Campos-Vega et al., (2010) described the changes in gene expression profiles in HT-29 colon cancer cells when exposed to specific fermented extract (FE) from common bean cv. Bayo Madero. Seventy-two genes were differentially expressed in HT-29 cells treated with FE (Figures 2 and 3). The authors found that SIAH1 gene was up-regulated, while p53 and RB were down-regulated, suggesting that the FE may be involved in the induction of G1-S cycle arrest. Furthermore, p21, p16 and cyclin B2 were up-regulated, whereas Cdk1 and cyclin E2 were down regulated by FE, indicating their potential role on G2-M cycle arrest induction. Finally, FE modulated genes involved in triggering apoptosis such as Bax, Bcl-2 and Tnfrsf10b. The effects of FE from common beans on HT-29 colon cancer cells were associated with short chain fatty acids, mainly butyrate, produced by *in vitro* fermentation (Campos-Vega et al., 2009). There is very extensive evidence from *in vitro* studies that butyrate may be antineoplastic, since it suppresses the growth of tumour cells and induces apoptosis (Hague et al., 1993). Microarray studies have been used to investigate the anticancer effects of butyrate on p53, p21, Rb, different Cyclins, E2F, and Histones, demonstrating a complex cascade of reprogramming in SW620 colonic epithelial cells upon treatment with butyrate. The reprogramming was also characterized by the progressive recruitment of gene sets as a function of time (Mariadason et al., 2000). In invasive human colonocytes, butyrate was the most potent inhibitor of PCNA, a clinically useful marker of cancer proliferation (Emenaker et al., 2001).

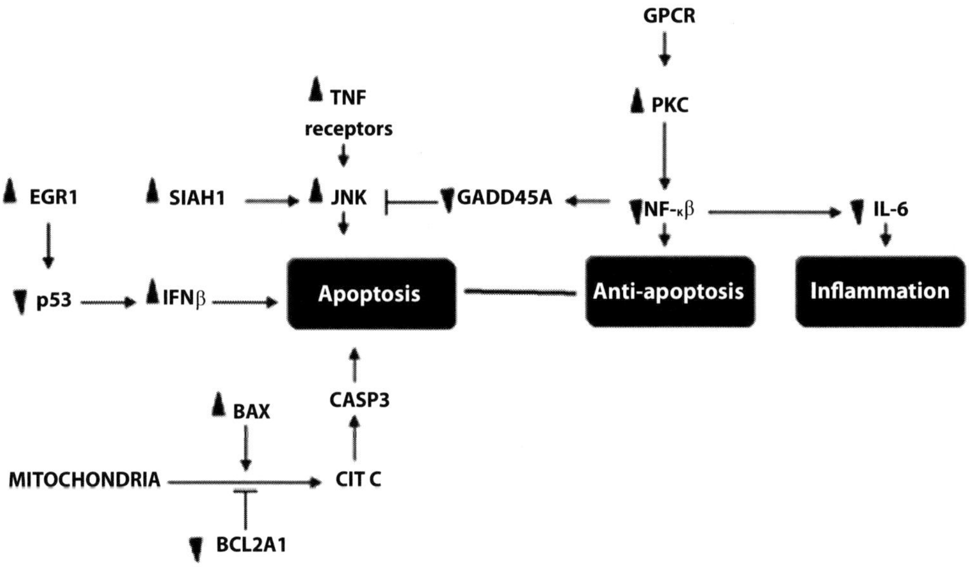

Figure 2. Changes in gene expression in apoptosis and inflammatory pathways. Symbols indicate up-regulation (▲) or down regulation (▼) in mRNA expression as derived from array analysis (Adapted from Campos-Vega et al, 2010).

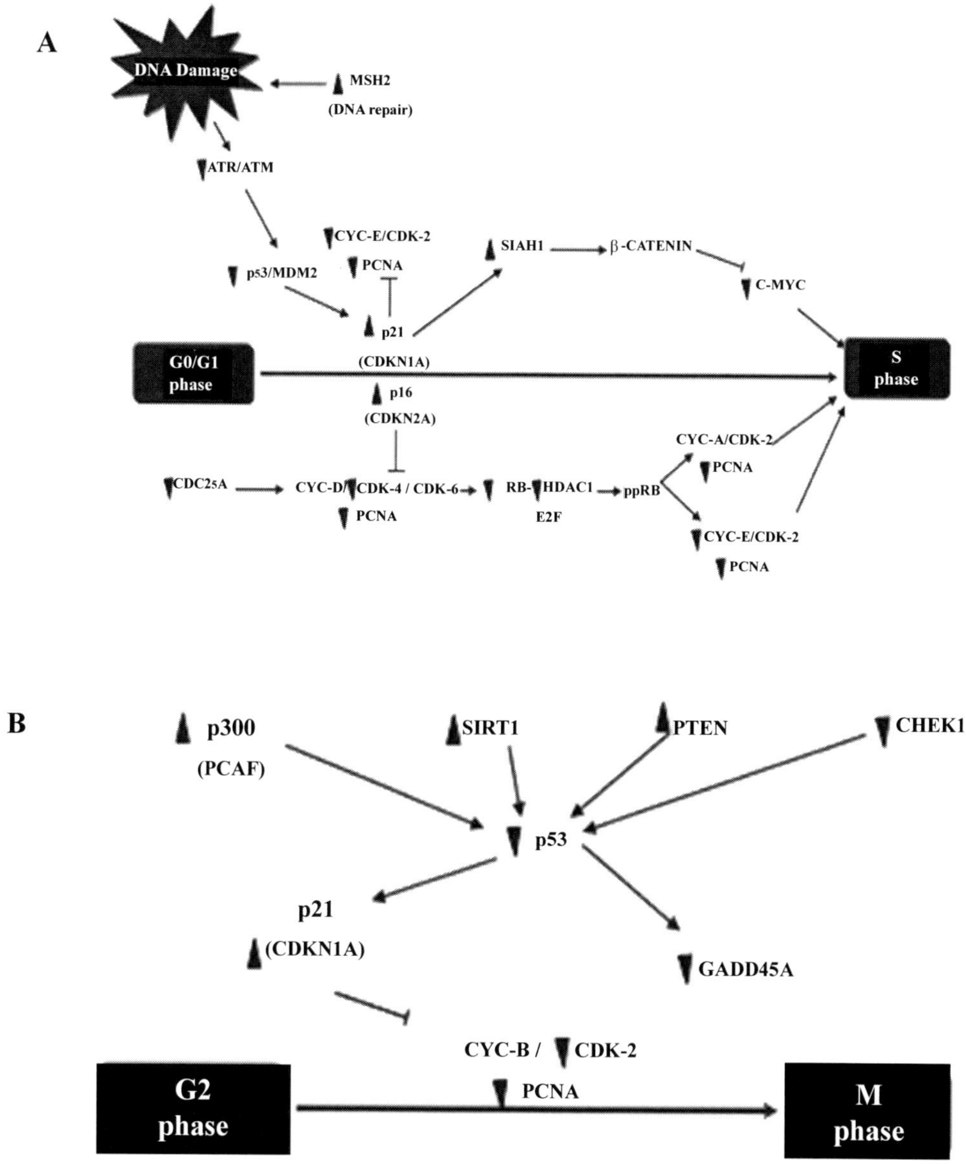

Figure 3. Changes in gene expression in G1/S (A) and G2/M (B) cell cycle phases. Symbols indicate up-regulation (▲) or down regulation (▼) in mRNA expression as derived from array analysis (Adapted from Campos-Vega et al, 2010).

Also, pulses are useful sources of many micronutrients (Se and Zn) and non-nutrient bioactive substances (phytates) which may improve antioxidant defenses (Mathers, 2002).

Significant antioxidant activities and phenolic compounds in several commonly consumed pulses have been reported (Smulikowska et al., 2001; Cardador-Martinez et al., 2002; Beninger and Hosfield 2003; Aparicio-Fernández et al., 2005; Espinosa-Alonso et al., 2006; Campos-Vega et al., 2009; Vergara-Castañeda et al., 2010).

Specifically, it has been reported that common beans contain total phenolic compounds (0.57-6.99 mg of GAE/g), flavonoids (0.92 to 4.24 mg of CAE/g) and condensed tannins (0.47 to 5.73 mg of CAE/g) in several cultivars with different seed coat colors (black, white, pinto, red, pink) (Xu et al., 2007). The effect of phenolic compounds from common beans on different diseases has been studied as an effort to prevent the development of such diseases and/or to create legume-based formulations that improve health.

The global scientific research has focused its effort on studying the effect of soybean on gene expression, trying to prevent and/or treat different diseases. But, in fact the phenolic composition in pulses and soybean is very similar, so it can be suggested that the modulation of molecular pathways may be similar to both seeds. The extract from black soybeans significantly reduced gene expression of TNF-α, MCP-1, and IL-6 in mesenteric adipose tissue, as reported by Kanamoto et al., (2011), concluding that the extract has the potential to ameliorate the inflammatory responses accompanying obesity. Suppression of the inflammatory state by black soybean extract may lead to reduced risk of cardiovascular diseases and atherosclerosis. The authors propose that cyanidin 3-glucoside, catechin and procyanidins possess beneficial actions independently against obesity, glucose intolerance, inflammation, and up-regulation of UCPs. As mentioned above, common bean has varying amounts of the same phenolic compounds, depending on the seed coat color (Gálvez-Ranilla, 2007). Therefore, it is important to note that the effects may be similar to those determined by these authors.

The flavonoid cyanidin 3-glucoside (Cy-3-G) extracted from black beans significantly promoted the mRNA expressions of peroxisome proliferrator-activated receptor-g (PPARγ), CCAAT/enhancer binding protein α (C/EBPα), and glucose transport 4 (GLUT4) in differentiated 3T3-L1 cells. Cy-3-G promotes adipocyte differentiation and uptake of glucose in a dose-dependent manner, significantly reduces TNF-α concentration and ROS production, and increases the adiponectin concentration in differentiated 3T3-L1 cell in a dose-dependent manner. These effects suggest that Cy-3-G would contribute to the improvement of insulin resistance and its consequences (Han et al., 2012; Inaguma et al., 2011).

Recently, plant polyphenols were reported to potentially suppress the vascular expression of nicotinamide adenine dinucleotide phosphate (NADPH) oxidase subunits (Sarr et al., 2006; Sanchez et al., 2006). Excessive production of reactive oxygen species (ROS), such as superoxide ($O2^-$), causes oxidative stress in the renal and vascular tissues (Guzik et al., 2000; Taniyama et al., 2003; Cuzzocrea et al., 2004). $O2^-$ is produced by various enzymes, particularly by NADPH oxidase, in the endothelium and smooth muscle cells of the arteries. Excess $O2^-$ forms peroxynitrite ($ONOO^-$), interacting with inducible nitric oxide synthase (iNOS)-derived nitric oxide (NO), and induces endothelial dysfunction and change in vascular response (Kumar et a., 2005; Alvarez et al., 2008). In this regard, polyphenol extracted from bean seed coats has been assessed on the attenuation of vascular oxidative stress and/or inflammation during the progression of hypertension, and this may lead to an improvement in hypertension. Mukai and Sato (2011) investigated the effects of azuki bean (*Vigna angularis*) seed coats (ABSC), which contain polyphenols, on the vascular oxidative stress and inflammation associated with hypertension in spontaneously hypertensive rats (SHR). The authors found that ABSC attenuated vascular $O2^-$ production by down-regulation of NADPH oxidase subunits, and suppressed the expression of iNOS, COX-2 and MCP-1/CCR2 in the aorta of SHR. In conclusion, these beans should be useful as a preventive strategy for atherosclerosis. Oomah et al., (2010) also indicated that bean hull water extracts were stronger inhibitors of lipoxygenase (15-LOX). These authors concluded that bean hull polyphenolics exert strong antiinflammatory effects even outperforming aspirin and that anti-inflammatory activity of bean hulls was dependent on their phenolic content and antioxidant activity that were significantly affected by cultivar and extracting solvent.

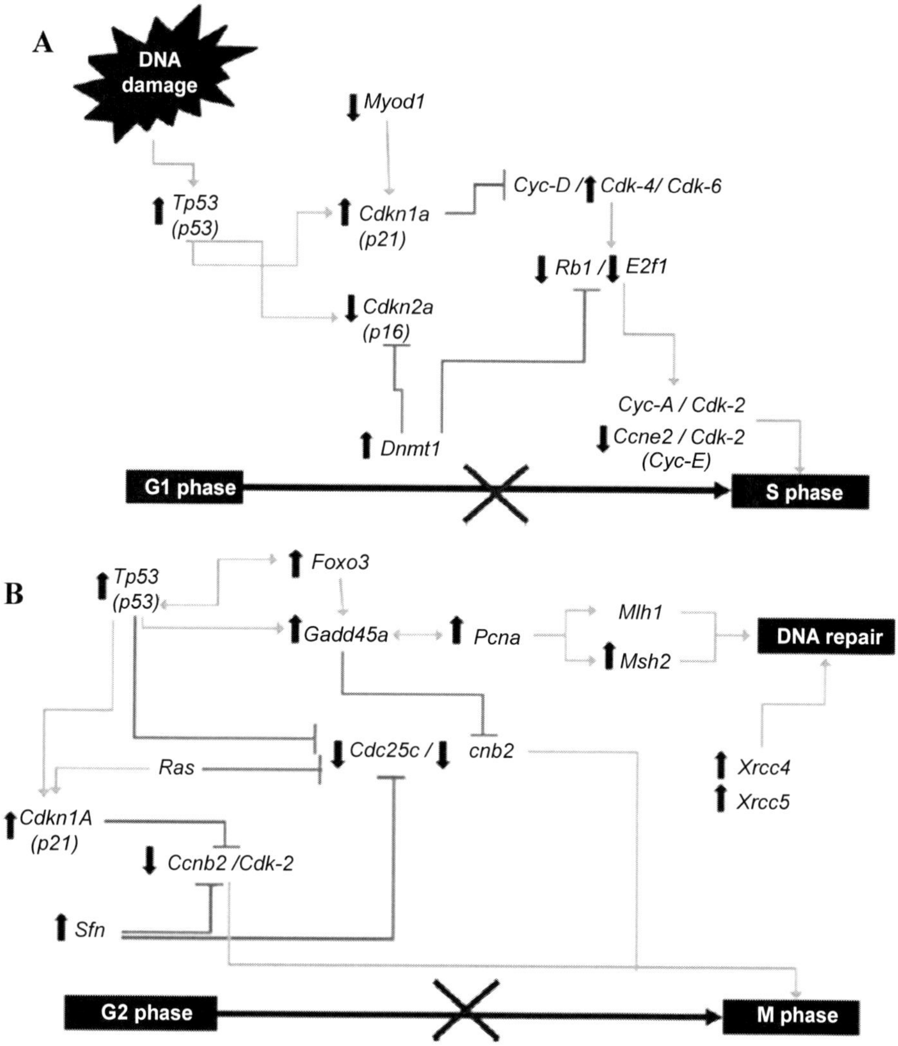

Figure 4. Changes in gene expression in G1/S (A) and G2/M (B) cell cycle phases. Symbols indicate up-regulation (▲) or down regulation (▼) in mRNA expression as derived from array analysis (Adapted from Campos-Vega et al, 2010).

Bean fiber contributes to the improvement of serum lipid levels; however other compounds such as phenolics may also contribute to this effect. Finley et al., (2007) showed that pinto bean consumption lowered serum total, HDL- and LDL-cholesterols, without affecting serum triglycerides, VLDL cholesterol, or glucose in adults with premetabolic syndrome. That study provided evidence that bean consumption can improve lipid profiles associated with cardiovascular disease. However, more notable finding of this study was the lack of changes in fermentation of the fiber from pinto beans. Thus, the authors concluded that perhaps the dietary fiber/fermentation hypothesis has been overstated and many of the real health benefits of eating beans are from components of beans not associated with fermentation. Many clinical, animal, and *in vitro* studies have reported the lipid-modifying effects of dietary phenolics from various preparations and extracts made from other foods (Auger et al., 2005; Castilla et al., 2006; Covas et al., 2006; Davalos et al., 2006).

Furthermore, the phenolic compounds in synergy with other constituents of bean seeds also participate in the prevention of cancer development through the modulation of gene expression. Vergara-Castañeda et al., (2012) evaluated the protective effect of non-digestible fraction (NDF) from common beans Bayo Madero cultivar on AOM-induced rats by PCR array. NDF contained mainly phenolic compounds, oligosaccharides, resistant starch and presumably biopeptides. The results indicated that Tp53, Gadd45a, Cdkn1a and Bax were highly expressed by NDF, whereas Cdc25c, Ccne2, E2f1 and Bcl2 were significantly suppressed, among others genes, compared to AOM group, suggesting that chemoprevention of NDF results from a combination of cell cycle arrest at G1/S and G2/M phases and cell death by apoptotic induction. NDF also increased the expression of Xrcc4, Xrcc and PCNA, suggesting its participation on DNA repair (Figures 4 and 5).

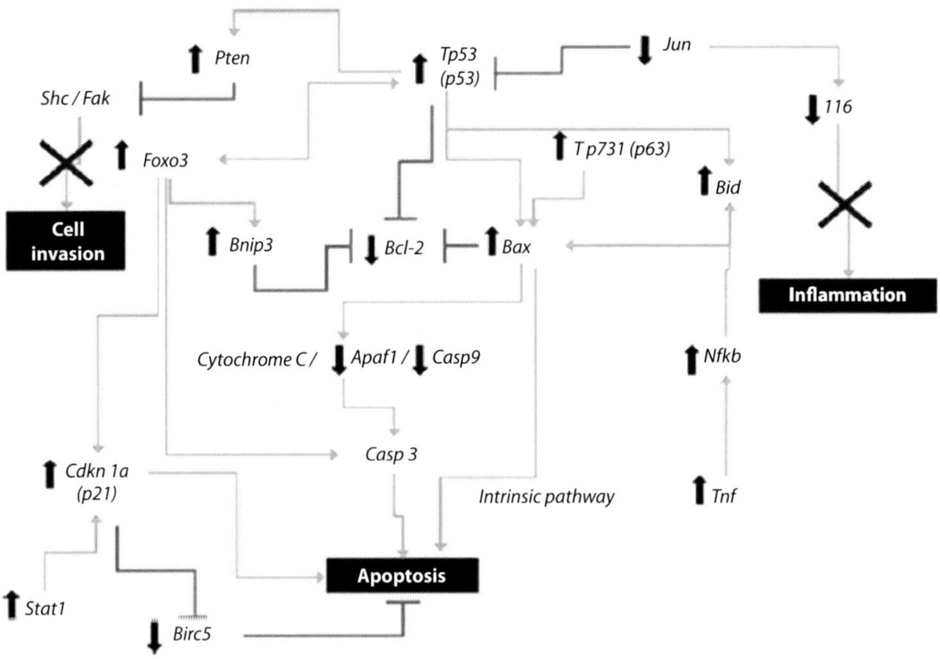

Figure 5. Changes in gene expression in apoptosis and inflammatory pathways. Symbols indicate up-regulation (⬆) and down-regulation (⬇) in mRNA expression as derived from array analysis, and signalling pathway interruption (✖) (Adapted from Vergara-Castañeda et al, 2012).

The protective effect of common beans on cancer development has been observed on several cell lines. The methanol extract from Jamapa beans, which contains condensed tannins and anthocyanins, inhibited HeLa (human cervix adenocarcinoma) cell proliferation in a dose-dependent manner. This extract affected HaCaT (human premalignant keratinocytic cells) used as non-cancerous control, to a lesser extent (Aparicio-Fernández et al., 2006). The inhibition on cell proliferation results from an increase in the expression of Bax and Caspase-3 proteins in HeLa cells by the methanol extract from Jamapa beans so, the apoptotic induction in HeLa cells is triggered mainly by the mitochondrial pathway (Aparicio-Fernández et al., 2008).

Isoflavones from pulses, structurally similar to estrogens, interact with estrogen receptors and may decrease serum cholesterol concentrations by similar mechanisms (Anderson, 1996). Isoflavones could bind to the ligand-binding domain of the estrogen receptor (ER), thereby initiating a series of molecular events culminating in several classical estrogen responses such as the induction of the progesterone receptor (PR) gene (Mueller, 2002), interfering with steroid hormone metabolism or action (Adlercreutz, 1998) and altering ER structure and affecting transcription (Santti et al., 1998; Po et al., 2002). *In vitro* studies of vascular cell cultures have shown that the isoflavone genistein inhibits atherosclerotic lesion development by inhibiting cell adhesion, altering growth factor activity, and inhibiting cell proliferation (Raines et al., 1995; Fotsis et al., 1995). Daidzein acts as an agonist for both ERα and ERβ and induces ER-mediated estrogenic responses both *in vitro* (Kaldas and Hughes, 1989) and *in vivo* (Baird et al., 2005; Hargreaves et al., 1999; Setchell et al., 2002). Daidzein has much lower affinity than genistein for binding to and transactivation through ERα and ERβ (Sathyamoorthy and Wang, 1997).

In earlier studies using differential display of mRNA and macroarrays, it was demonstrated that soy protein diets containing different levels of isoflavone have variable effects on changes in gene expression in female obese Zucker rats. By combining ddmRNA and macroarray analysis, genes involved in lipid metabolism, regulation of transcription and translation, protease inhibition, apoptosis, and cell proliferation regulation were found to be expressed at higher levels in rat livers fed with the low-isoflavone soy protein and high-isoflavone soy protein diet compared with the liver of control diet animals. The coordinated regulation of these genes in liver further supports the hypothesis of multiple health benefits of isoflavones in synergy with other compounds (Iqbal et al., 2002).

Although common bean is not recognized as an isoflavone source as soybean, several authors have found considerable amounts of these isoflavones in some bean varieties. During germination of seven common beans seed samples, daidzein (8.2 to 129.1 μg/g), genistein (2.6 to 9.7 μg/g), and coumestrol (2.4 to 35.6 μg/ g) were identified (Espinosa-Alonso et al., 2006). Díaz-Batalla et al., (2006) also quantified quercetin, kaempferol, daidzein, genistein, coumestrol and phenolic acid contents in 72-h-germinated Mexican common bean seeds.

The study of Zhao et al., (2007) shows that extracts of Adzuki bean and Lima bean could alter the intracellular distribution of estrogen receptor (ER) via different patterns. Lima bean extracts exhibited the same pattern as that of E2, while Adzuki bean extracts up-regulated the ER in cytoplasm, with no decrease observed in nuclear ER expression. Both, Adzuki bean and Lima bean extracts, showed the same effects on progesterone receptor mRNA and protein expression, the results strongly suggested that different interaction patterns with the estrogen receptor were involved in their estrogen-like activities.

Bioactive peptides arising from diet proteins may be present as independent entities or encoded in the original protein, and they are released from precursor proteins during digestion or food processing (Vioque et al., 2006). These peptides display several biological activities such as antihypertensive, opioid, antioxidant, anticholesterolemic, antimicrobial, anticariogenic, antithrombotic, anticancer and immunomodulatory (Torruco-Uco et al., 2008). The anticarcinogenic activity of some peptides released from food is due to their capacity to arrest cell cycle and induce apoptosis by Caspase-3 activation, topoisomerase-2 inihibition or NFkB reduction and interleukin-6 activation (González de Mejía and Prisecaru, 2005; Torruco-Uco et al., 2009). Even when these peptides have mainly been studied in soybean, amaranth and other cereals, recent interest has led to their identification and characterization in common beans. Torruco-Uco et al., (2009) hydrolyzed Mexican common bean (*Phaseolus vulgaris* L.) seeds, cv. Jamapa, with different enzymes, obtaining peptides of low molecular weight (13-26.5 kDa). The hydrolysates exhibited antioxidant activity determined by ABTS assay. García-Gasca et al., (2002) evaluated the antiproliferative effect of a protein fraction from tepary bean (*Phaseolus acutifolius*) seeds with protease inhibitory activity (TPIF), on normal and on malignant cells. They reported that, although proliferation of epithelial HeLa cells (malignant cells) were not affected by TPIF, fibroblastic transformed cells were highly affected in a dose-dependent ratio.

Beans contain other proteins with biological activity such as as lectins and hemagglutinins. Both are bioactive proteins or glycoproteins that agglutinate erythrocytes of some or all blood groups *in vitro* depending on their specificity and high binding affinity for a particular carbohydrate moiety on the cell surface. Lectins can bind to glycoprotein receptors on cell membranes; this binding is necessary for cell agglutination (González De Mejía and Prisecaru, 2005). Lectins and hemagglutinins are mostly found in seeds, especially from legumes seeds (Lam and Ng, 2011). Bean lectins reduce the growth of non-Hodgkin's lymphoma (Pryme et al., 1999) and can screen serum samples from patients with pancreatic cancer or pancreatitis by selective detection of glycan structures (Harland, 2002).

Raw common bean and bean globulins contain high amounts of lectins (820 and 1640 HU/mg of dry matter in raw common bean and globulins, respectively) (Carbonaro et al., 2000). Lectin content in 19 varieties of *Phaseolus vulgaris* from Spain ranged from 1.89 to 9.99 g/kg (Muzquiz et al., 1999). Bayo Victoria, a Durango race cultivar, had three times more lectins than levels reported for soybean (González de Mejia et al., 2003). Activity of common bean lectin is 8573 U/mg protein (González de Mejía et al., 2005), but other common beans may contain 20 g of lectin per 100 g of flour (Burbano et al., 1999). Barampama and Simard (1993) reported lectin content for four varieties of dry beans *Phaseolus vulgaris* L (A321, A410, Calima and Dore de Kirundo) cultivated in different regions, with hemagglutinin activity units (HAU) from 0.42 to 8.89 HAU/g (average 2.15 HAU/g). González de Mejia et al., (2005) reported that HAU from common bean (*Phaseolus vulgaris* cultivar Flor de Mayo) and tepary beans (*Phaseolus acutifolius*, white, black and brown cultivars) inhibited the viability on rat epithelial cells (expressed as percent of cellularity) and was significantly different among protein extracts from different bean cultivars. Common bean extract showed the lowest cytotoxicity (87.4% cellular viability).

The hemagglutinin from *Phaseolus vulgaris* cv. *Legumi secchi* potently inhibits the proliferation of human breast cancer cells. Low concentration of hemagglutinin that produced half of the cells underwent the early phase of apoptosis. Exposure to higher hemagglutinin concentrations resulted in 88% shift of the cell population from normal to the early/late apoptotic/necrotic stage. *Legumi Secchi* hemagglutinin-treated MCF-7 cells exhibits phosphatidylserine externalisation and mitochondrial membrane depolarisation. As the concentration of the hemagglutinin increased, the expression of Fas, caspase-8, truncated BID, p53, and truncated Lamin A/C increased in a dose-dependent manner. Flow cytometry analysis revealed that more MCF-7 cells displayed mitochondrial membrane depolarization when the hemagglutinin concentration was raised (Lam and Ng, 2011).

PEAS

Around 20 leguminous species are used as dry grains in appreciable amounts for human nutrition. Among these, pea (*Pisum sativum* L.) is highly consumed in Asian countries. It is one of the four most important cultivated legumes alongside soybean, groundnut and beans (Morrow, 1991). Peas are found in two general varieties: sweet or green peas, and field pea. Field peas, also known as cowpeas or gray peas are the domesticated *Pisum sativum*. These are called "gray" due to the color of the seed and the flour they produce when ground. Field peas are harvested on the vine and dried for use. In contrast to wild peas, field peas typically maintain shorter, stronger vines (Weaver, 2003).

Peas are significant sources of protein, fiber, and many vitamins and minerals. As dry beans, peas also provide complex carbohydrates and soluble fiber. Peas contain 21.9% and 23.7% protein, 2.4% and 2.65% lipids,52.5% and 58.6% carbohydrate in raw and cooked peas, respectively and 3.4% ash (de Almeida Costa et al., 2006). The different types of carbohydrates in peas have been studied. Peas contain 42.2% starch, 3.5% soluble nonstarch polysaccharides, 12.9 and 3.7% of insoluble nonstarch polysaccharides and insoluble/soluble nonstarch polysaccharides fraction, respectively, and 16.4% of total soluble nonstarch polysaccharides. Moreover, oligosaccharides in peas consist of 0.03% glucose, 1.3% sucrose and 5.3% raffinose (Adamidou et al., 2011). Peas are an extremely low-fat food; the type of fat and fat-soluble nutrients they contain is impressive. Green peas are a reliable source of omega-3 fats in the form of alpha-linolenic acid (ALA).

Among micronutrients, peas have high ascorbic acid, β-carotene, thiamine and riboflavin contents and, compared with other vegetables, they are rich in iron (20.2 μg^{-1} of the edible portion) (Cabrera et al., 2003).

The content of ascorbic acid in peas ranging from 0.40 to 1.48 mmol/g (Doblado et al., 2005) was positively correlated with the total antioxidant capacity of the water-soluble compounds. In the study of Moriyama and Oba (Nilsson et al., 2004), the average value of total vitamin C per 100 g of dry weight in dehydrated samples was 4.14 mg in green peas present predominantly as dehydroascorbic acid. Peas, similar to beans, lentils and chickpeas, are also good sources of folate, the vitamin that lowers the blood level of homocysteine. High levels of homocysteine are associated with an increased risk of heart disease (Newgent, 2001).

Nutraceutical Properties of Peas

Some researchers have now speculated that the association between green pea and legume intake and lowered risk of type 2 diabetes may be connected not only with the relatively low glycemic index of green peas (about 45-50) and their strong fiber and protein content, but also with this unusual combination of antioxidant and anti-inflammatory phytonutrients.

Peas have considerably lower glycemic index values relative to other high-carbohydrate foods (Foster-Powell and Miller, 1995). Glycemic load is thought to be more important as an indicator of overall glycemic response because it takes into account both the quality (glycemic index) and quantity of carbohydrate (Davis et al., 2004).

Marinangeli et al., (2011) evaluated the effects of whole and fractionated yellow peas on circulating lipids, glucose and insulin levels, energy expenditure, and body composition, as well as their prebiotic effects in Golden Syrian hamsters. Consumption of whole pea flour (WPF), and fractionated pea flour (hulls only) (FPF) produced negligible effects on circulating cholesterol and triglyceride levels. However, both WPF and FPF reduced circulating insulin levels compared with the control group. Moreover, the authors found that FPF decreased circulating glucose levels compared with control group. Hamsters consuming WPF demonstrated higher oxygen consumption vs. the control group. Finally, the analysis of caecal digesta showed that WPF produced shifts in the abundance of microbial taxa with the most predominant changes occurring within the phylum Firmicutes. Therefore, yellow peas and their constituents could help prevent lifestyle-related diseases such as diabetes and obesity. In addition to its hypoglycemic and insulin effects, peas have significant hypocholesterolemic action, which could contribute to atherosclerosis prevention, and genes involved in this protection have recently been identified. Pea protein has low methionine and high arginine content and the arginine: lysine ratio is much higher than in casein. It has been suggested that the high arginine: lysine ratio may be responsible, at least partly, for the hypocholesterolemic effect of soy protein (Gudbrandsen et al., 2006). These similarities in the amino acid profile give rise to the fact that pea protein could exert similar effects on lipid metabolism as soy or lupin protein. A diet based on pea protein may decrease concentrations of cholesterol in VLDL and in the liver of rats. Additionally, pea protein diet increase the amount of bile acids excreted via faeces. Rats fed pea protein have higher relative mRNA concentrations of sterol regulatory element-binding protein (SREBP)-2, 3-hydroxy-3-methylglutaryl-CoA (HMG-CoA) reductase, LDL receptor and CYP7A1 (a key enzyme of hepatic bile acid synthesis) in the liver than rats fed a diet containing casein (Figure 6) (Spielmann et al., 2007).

Rigamonti et al., (2010) evaluated the hypolipidemic properties of pea proteins in an animal model. Plasma total cholesterol concentrations in rats fed pea protein isolate was significantly decreased. HDL cholesterol tended to be higher than in control rats and the pea protein-containing diet reduced triglyceride levels. The authors examining possible mechanisms for the pea protein mediated alterations of cholesterolemia, found that pea proteins significantly increased mRNA levels of the LDL receptor, the major regulator of circulating LDL cholesterol compared with control. The relative concentration of the transcription factor SREBP-1c in the liver as well as hepatic mRNA concentrations of FAS, SCD1 and SCD2 tended to be lower in the group fed pea proteins. The results of this study indicate that pea proteins exert a hypotriglyceridemic activity mainly through downregulation of fatty acid synthesis.

Protein intake may also have other beneficial effects associated with weight loss (Eisenstein et al., 2002). This effect has been attributed to the greater satiating potential of proteins compared to other macronutrients (Anderson and Moore, 2004; Westerterp-Plantengav, 2003). The source of protein may play a role in its satiating effect; however, inconsistent data exists from human studies. Recently, several foods have been shown to enhance satiety and decrease energy intake when consumed, resulting in higher weight loss during energy restriction (Luhovyy et al., 2007; Veldhorst et al., 2009; Vander et al., 2005). Abou-Samra et al., (2011) recently reported that pea protein is effective in lowering short term food intake. But, when the preload was consumed 30 min before the *ad libitum* meal, total food intake was similar after pea protein compared to after water control, with a caloric compensation of around 100%. Mechanisms were not explored but gastric emptying might play a role. Other potential mechanisms can be related to the action of satiety hormones. On the other hand, the pea protein preload administered as a starter before the meal did not lower *ad libitum* food intake. Furthermore, total intake was higher compared to the water control.

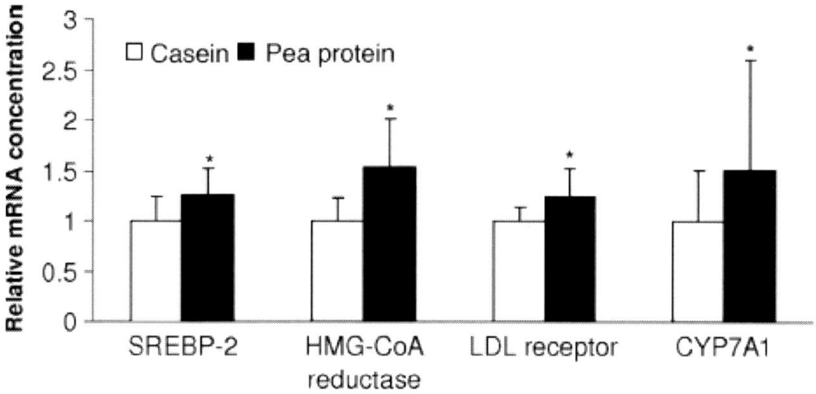

Figure 6. Relative mRNA concentrations of sterol regulatory element binding protein (SREBP)-2, 3-hydroxy-3-methylglutaryl coenzyme A (HMG-CoA)-reductase, LDL receptor and cholesterol 7α-hydroxylase (CYP7A1) in the liver of male rats fed diets containing 200 g/kg of casein or pea protein for 16 days. Values were related to the reference gene glyceraldehyde-3-phosphate-dehydrogenase (GAPDH). Each bar represents mean ± SD, n = 12. *Significantly different from rats fed the casein-based diet (=1.0), $p < 0.05$ (Adapted from Spielmann et al., 2007).

Food ingestion triggers many stimuli, such as the release of the gastrointestinal hormones cholecystokinin (CCK), glucagonlike peptide 1 (GLP-1) and peptide YY (PYY). These hormones are involved in the modulation of appetite sensations. Considering this fact, Geraedts et al., (2011) evaluated whether pea protein may alter hormone release, comparing the method of administration, between intraduodenal and oral in both lean and obese subjects. This study demonstrated for the first time that in both lean and obese humans, intraduodenal administration of intact pea protein is effective in reducing food intake, whereas no differences between placebo and treatment were observed after oral administration of the protein. They observed elevated levels of CCK in obese subjects and of GLP-1 and PYY in both groups (lean and obese subjects) after intraduodenal administration. This suggests that preventing gastric pea protein degradation may be an effective dietary strategy in the prevention and treatment of obesity. Another study showed that the combination of pea protein with sucrose and the artificial sweetener sucralose induced stronger effects on GLP-1 release both *in vitro* and *ex vivo* compared to the compounds separately. It was also shown that addition of sucrose or sucralose to STC-1 cells stimulated the release of CCK and GLP-1, whereas addition of the sweeteners to human duodenal biopsies did not result in hormone release. The conclusion of this study was that the combination of food ingredients plays an important role in the regulation of the release of satiety hormones (Geraedts et al., 2012).

More studies are necessary to conclude the beneficial effect of several types of proteins, as those of peas, on satiety. However, these studies suggest a possible involvement of peas on satiety, which may help in a major public health problem worldwide, such as obesity in both adults and children and its complications.

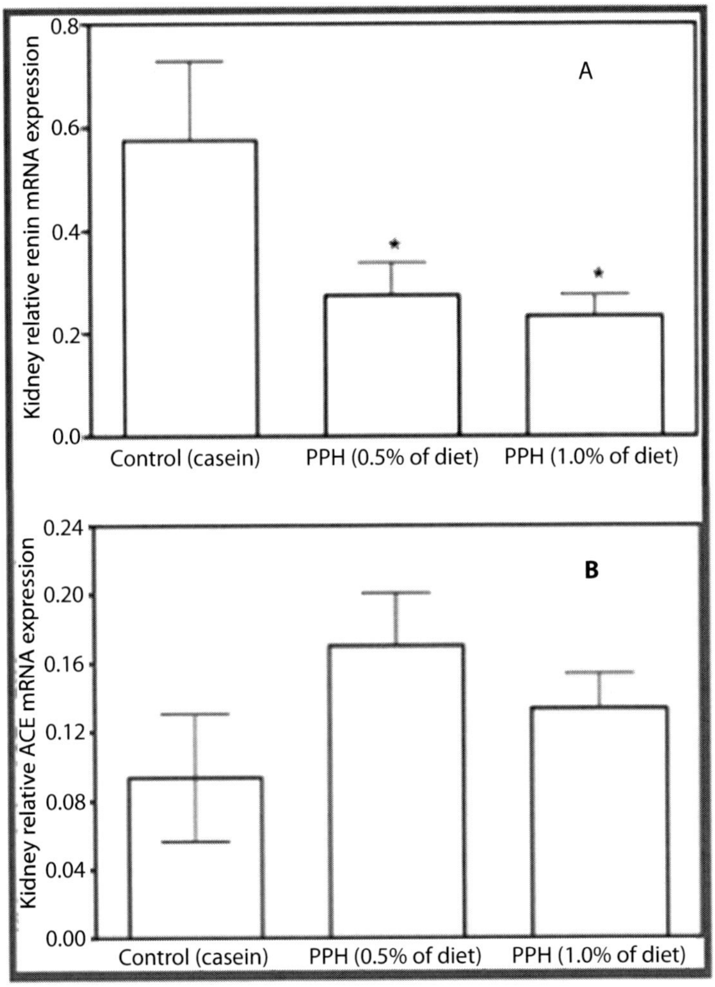

Figure 7. Effect of pea protein hydrolysate (PPH) on renal tissue level of renin (A) and angiotensin converting enzyme, ACE (B) mRNA in Han: SPRD-cy rats. Diets were formulated to contain 20% protein (casein) in the control rats but partially substituted with PPH (19.5% casein + 0.5% PPH or 19% casein + 1% PPH) in treated rats. *Significantly different from casein at $p < 0.05$ (Adapted from Li et al., 2011).

Rapid advances in biomedical research have revealed that certain proteins and their hydrolytic products such as Angiotensin I converting enzyme (ACE)-inhibitory peptides may possess regulatory activities and can be useful in the prevention and/or treatment of certain diseases (Meisel, 1997; FitzGerald et al., 2004). ACE inhibitory peptides may result in a lowering of the blood pressure by inhibition of the ACE enzyme, which results in decrease of the vasoconstrictor angiotensin II and increase in the vasodilator bradykinin (Eriksson et al., 2002). ACE inhibitory peptides have already been found in several food protein hydrolysates and ferments (Yamamoto 1997; Dziuba et al., 1999). Recent reports have shown isolation of three pea protein-derived peptides that had *in vitro* inhibitory activities against ACE and rennin (Fujita et al., 2000). Vermeirssen et al., (2005) studied the inhibitory action against ACE by pea proteins after intravenous administration of 50 mg/kg protein BW in spontaneously hypertensive rats (SHR), and the result was that pea digest exerted a transient, but strong antihypertensive effect of 44.4 mmHg. They found that ACE inhibitory peptides in pea permeate, with high stability to peptidases, could exert a transient antihypertensive effect before being broken down in the plasma. These results suggest that pea digest could be a promising source of ACE inhibitory peptides for use in the prevention and treatment of hypertension.

Li et al., (2011) also reported that pea protein hydrolysate (PPH) showed weak *in vitro* activities against renin and angiotensin converting enzyme (ACE) with inhibitory activities of 17 and 19%, respectively, at 1 mg/mL test concentration (Figure 7). Oral administration of the PPH to spontaneously hypertensive rats (SHR) at 100 and 200 mg/kg body weight lowered the hourly systolic blood pressure (SBP), with a maximum reduction of 19 mmHg at 4 h. In contrast, orally administered unhydrolyzed PPI had no blood pressure reducing effect in SHR, suggesting that thermolysin hydrolysis may have been responsible for releasing bioactive peptides from the native protein. Oral administration of PPH to the Han: SPRD-cy rat (a model of chronic kidney disease) over an 8-week period led to 29 and 25 mmHg reductions in SBP and diastolic blood pressure, respectively. The PPH-fed rats had lower plasma levels of angiotensin II but there was no effect on plasma activity or renal mRNA levels of ACE. However, renal expression of renin mRNA levels was reduced by approximately 50% in the PPH-fed rats, suggesting that reduced renin may be responsible for the reduced levels of angiotensin II. These results are important because cardiovascular complications, including hypertension, are often associated with CKD and are the most common cause of fatality (Sarnak et al., 2003).

Murakami et al., (2001b) evaluated the hepatoprotective effect of the flavonol oligoglycosides from *P. sativum* in primary cultured mouse hepatocytes, and found that quercetin 3-sophorotrioside, a principal constituent, exerted inhibitory effect, but the activities of other compounds were very weak.

On the other hand, carotenoids, in view of their antioxidant properties have received considerable interest by researchers, health professionals and regulatory agencies. In plants, they contribute to the photosynthetic machinery and protect against photo-damage, and in human, they are important in preventing diseases including cardiovascular diseases, cancer and other chronic diseases (Astrog et al., 1997; Rao and Rao, 2007). Based on epidemiological studies a positive link has been suggested between higher dietary intake and tissue concentrations of carotenoids and lower risk of chronic diseases (Johnson, 2002). The antioxidant properties of carotenoids have been proposed as the main mechanism by which they afford their beneficial effects (Agarwal and Rao, 2000). The principal carotenoids of foods are β-carotene, β-cryptoxanthin, lycopene, lutein and violaxanthin (Dutta et al., 2005). Several cultivars of peas have considerable carotenoid content.

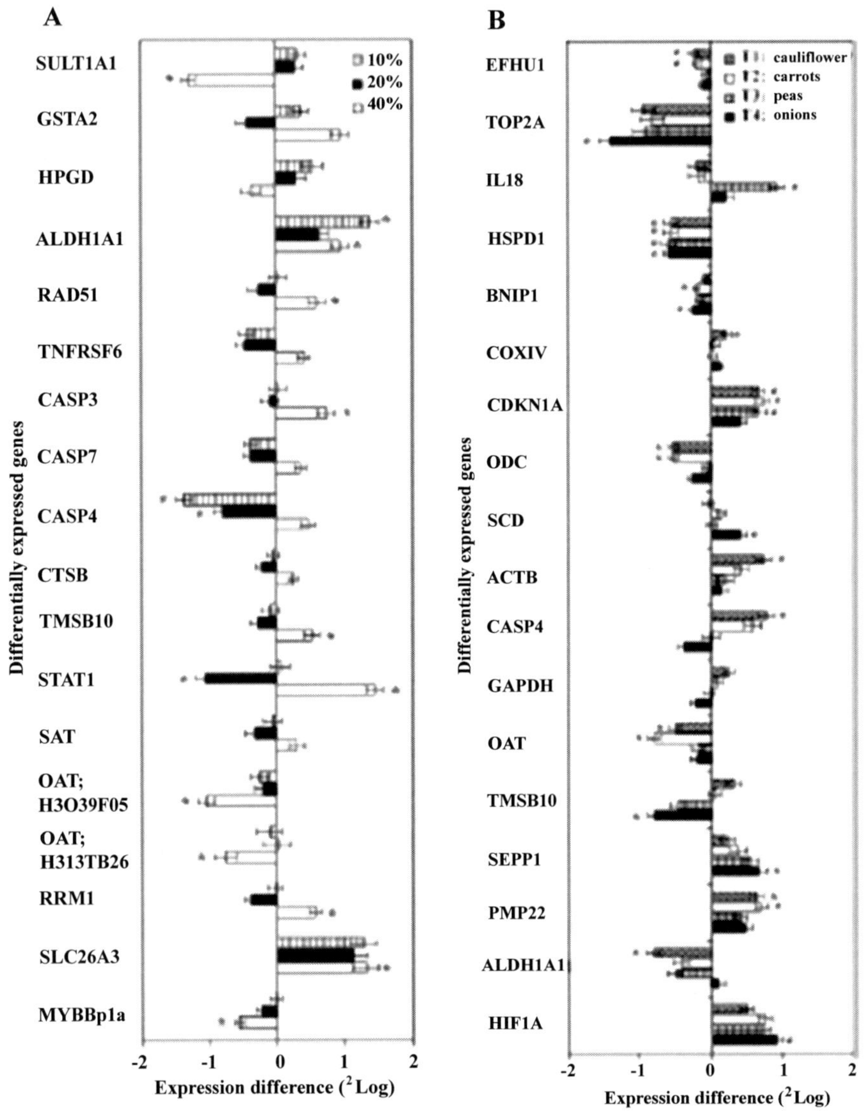

Figure 8. Gene expression differences in the colon mucosa of female C57Bl/6 mice fed different vegetable diets for 2 wk. (*A*) Expression profiles of the genes (SULT1A1, GSTA2, HPGD, ALDH1A1, RAD51, TNFRSF6, CASP3, CASP7, CASP4,CTSB, TMSB10, STAT1, SAT, OAT, RRM1, SLC26A3, and MYBBp1a) likely to play a role at various stages of CRC development that were modulated by diets containing 10%, 20%, or 40% doses (wt:wt) of a vegetable mixture consisting of cauliflower, carrots, peas, and onions, compared to control (set to 0); (*B*) Expression profiles of all genes (EFHU1, TOP2A, IL18, HSPD1, BNIP1, COXIV, CDKN1A, ODC, SCD, ACTB, GAPDH, OAT, TMSB10, SEPP1, PMP22, ALDH1A1, and HIF1A) that were differentially expressed in one or more groups of mice fed diets containing individual vegetables (cauliflower, carrots, peas, or onions; dose equal to individual level in the 40%-dose vegetable-mixture diet), compared to control (set to 0). Values are estimated difference in mean 2log-transformed intensity ± SE per vegetable group compared to the control group (set to 0), $n = 3$. *Different from control group, $P < 0.0001$ (ANOVA, *P*-value after Bonferroni correction) (Adapted from Breda et al., 2005a).

One study conducted in six cultivars of processed green peas (Avola, Tristar, Rampart, Turon, Bella, and Greenshaft) identified 17 chlorophyll and carotenoid pigments including 8 xanthophylls [(*all-E*)-neoxanthin, (9'*Z*)-neoxanthin, (*all-E*)-violaxanthin, neochrome, (*all-E*)-lutein epoxide, (*all-E*)-lutein, neolutein B, neolutein A], 4 chlorophyll *b* related compounds (chlorophyll *b* derivative, chlorophyll *b*, chlorophyll *b*', and pheophytin *b*), 4 chlorophyll *a* related compounds (chlorophyll *a* derivative, chlorophyll *a*, chlorophyll *a*', and pheophytin *a*), and (*all-E*)-β-carotene. All the pigments increased with time (2 years) in the six cultivars probably in relation to maturity, product color and nutritional quality (Edelenbos et al., 2001). Also, Marles et al., (2012) found *trans*-lutein and chlorophylls *a* and *b in* mature hulls of yellow and green market classes of peas, while in developing hulls, violaxanthin, neoxanthin, lutein, zeaxanthin, chlorophylls*a* and *b* and β-carotene were detected.

Moreover, high consumption of carotenoid from fruit and vegetables are inversely associated with mortality for various cancers, including colon cancer. Specifically, Rijken et al., (1999) investigated the effect of consuming standard diets supplemented with freeze-dried vegetable, including peas and some carotenoids on surrogate end-point markers for colorectal cancer in an azoxymethane-induced rat model. The authors found that the mean multiplicity per focus in aberrant crypts was significantly reduced in the pea-supplemented diet, and the carotenoids inhibited aberrant crypt multiplicity only marginally. Van Breda et al., (2005a) investigated the effects of 4 vegetables (cauliflower, carrots, peas, and onions) on gene expression in the colonic mucosa of female C57Bl/6 mice using microarray technology. Heat shock 60 kDa protein 1 (chaperonin) (HSPD1) is the only gene expression modulated in all vegetable groups compared to the control group. HSPD1 encodes for a member of the family of chaperones, which can be defined as proteins assisting other proteins to reach their final active forms, maintaining the homeostasis, thereby reducing the call for stress-induced proteins, resulting in their decreased transcription (Garrido et al., 2001). Cyclin-dependent kinase inhibitor 1A (p21) (CDKNIA), which participates in apoptosis and cell cycle arrest (El-Deiry et al., 1993; Bunz et al., 1998), was affected by peas and interleukin 18 (interferon-gamma-inducing factor) gene expression was also up-regulated. IL18 encodes for a type-1 T-helper cytokine which has antitumour activities by increasing apoptosis (Marino and Cardier, 2003), inhibiting angiogenesis (Coughlin et al., 1998) and maintaining homeostasis (Pages et al., 1999). The modulation of these three genes (HSPD1, IL18 and CDKN1A) by peas is expected to increase colorectal cancer protective mechanisms (Figure 8).

Pea consumption in cancer development has also been investigated in other organs. Van Breda et al., (2005b) evaluated the effect of several vegetables, including peas, on gene expression changes in the lungs of female C57Bl/6 mice using cDNA microarray technology. Pea intake modulated the expression of three genes: hemoglobin α, adult chain 1 (HBA-A1) decreased while glutathione reductase 1 (GSR) and LDL receptor (LDLR) increased. GSR encodes for an enzyme that reduces oxidized glutathione involved in the antioxidative defense system against endogenous and exogenous prooxidants (Vang et al., 1997). This result is important because it demonstrate that vegetables induce GSR expression in the lungs, thereby probably supplementing the lungs with more reduced oxidized glutathione and possibly resulting in an improved antioxidative defense in the lungs. The protein product of LDLR is a cell surface receptor that plays an important role in cholesterol homeostasis. The authors showed that tumor cell lines have higher LDLR activity than the corresponding normal cells. Furthermore, LDL uptake was higher in lung tumor tissue than in the corresponding normal tissue. Two of the three genes modulated by peas may be involved in lung cancer preventive pathways; only the effect on GSR may lead to lung cancer risk prevention by inducing antioxidative defense.

Traka et al., (2010) compared changes in gene expression induced by sulforaphane in PTEN-null mice with previously reported changes in human prostate tissue following diets enriched in either broccoli (a dietary source of sulforaphane) or peas. They found evidence that both diets may induce similar changes. The authors suggested that in addition to sulforaphane derived from broccoli, some dietary component common to both diets may be able to suppress the downstream effects of PTEN deletion, possibly by lignans, such as secoisolariciresinol, and flavonoids which are present in both peas and broccoli, and which have been associated with reduction in prostate cancer risk (McCullough and Giovannucci, 2004; Khan et al., 2008). Lignans are converted by intestinal microflora to enterodiol and enterolactone, which have been shown to suppress pAKT expression in cell models (Chen et al., 2009) and certain flavonoids modulate PI3K/AKT signaling (Hou and Kumamoto, 2010).

In addition to carotenoids activity, the protector effect in different diseases could also be due to the action of other compounds present in pea seeds. It is clear that phenolic compounds have a potential beneficial effect through their antioxidant and antimutagenic activities. The phenolic extracts obtained from different foods present high antioxidant activity, determined by its capacity to bind free radicals and inhibit lipid peroxidation (Oomah et al., 2005; Amarowicz, 2007; Fresco et al., 2010). Biologically-active compounds of interest found in leguminous seeds come from many chemical classes and include phenolic acids as well as their derivatives, flavanols, flavan-3-ols, anthocyanins/anthocyanidins, condensed tannins/proanthocyanidins, tocopherols, and vitamin C (Amarowicz and Pegg, 2008).

Seeds and fruit rinds from *Pisum sativum* L. were studied for phenolic compounds and antimicrobial activity by Chanda et al., (2010). The authors report a total phenolic content of 6.84 mg gallic acid equivalents (GAE)/g in the ethyl acetate extract from seeds and 7.76 mg GAE/g in the same extract from the fruit rind. Methanolic extract of seeds and fruit rind contain 8.45 and 11.62 mg GAE/g total phenolics, while aqueous extract has almost similar content 11.12 and 11.26 mg GAE/g, respectively. Finally, the extracts of the seeds of *P. sativum* showed activity against *B. subtilis*. Marles et al., (2012) detected polyphenolics and hydroxybenzoic in 'dun' and 'maple' field pea types and the occurrence of flavonoid-related compounds was correlated only with pigmented seed coat genotypes.

Xu et al., (2007) reported the phenolic conent in different cultivars of yellow and green peas. Total phenolic content of ten yellow pea cultivars ranged from 0.85 mg to 1.14 mg GAE/g, while the range was 0.65 mg to 0.99 mg in ten green pea cultivars. The total flavonoid content of yellow pea cultivars ranged from 0.09 to 0.17 mg catechin equivalents/g, while condensed tannin content of yellow and green pea cultivars ranged from 0.22 to 0.61 mg catechin equivalents/g. These yellow and green pea cultivars exhibited radical DPPH scavenging activity, ferric reducing antioxidant power and oxygen radical absorbing capacity. Therefore, these cultivars are a good source of antioxidant compounds with potential biological activity. Thirty-five varieties of the green pea (*Pisum sativum* L.) were analyzed for their total antioxidant capacity (TAC). After blanching and freezing, the water-soluble and water-insoluble fractions had, on average, TAC of 0.61 and 0.23 μmol/g, respectively. Ascorbic acid accounted for a large part of the water-soluble antioxidant capacity (Nilsson et al., 2004). Moreover, the antioxidant activity of a pea extract and its fractions of low molecular phenolics and tannins have been evaluated using several assays. Amarowicz and Troszyñska (2003) reported that phenolic compounds present in extract and its fractions displayed antioxidant and antiradical properties, but the results of assays performed were the highest when tannins (fraction II) were tested. The effect of the extract on the couple oxidation of linoleic acid and β-carotene was highest than the two fractions. This extract contained vanillic, caffeic, *p*-coumaric and ferulic acids, sinapic, quercetin, kaempherol, procyanidin B2 and B3.. Total antioxidant activity of tannin fraction was 2.48 μmol Trolox/mg, whereas the extract and fraction I showed only 0.30 and 0.22 μmol Trolox/mg, respectively. The fraction II exhibited several times higher antiradical activity than crude extract and its low molecular phenolics fraction I tested by DPPH assay.

The presence of these compounds in peas is very important in the sense that is widely reported that phenolic compounds are involved in different molecular signaling pathways, through the modulation in expression of genes involved in proliferation, apoptosis, cell cycle arrest, inflammation, among others (Kuo, 1994; Richter et al., 1999; Chen et al., 2000; Yang et al., 2000; Hu and Kong, 2004). It can be suggested that phenolic compounds contained in pea seeds could have all of these activities to provide health benefits and achieve a state of wellness in people. In general, peas have not been as studied in preventing diseases as common bean consumption, but with the information presented in this chapter we can realize the impact that peas have on health, broad range of phytochemical constituents and the opportunities of research yet to be explored with this food trying to prevent the development of disease and improving the health of the population.

CHICKPEAS

Chickpeas is the third most important cool-season food legume after common bean (*Phaseolus vulgaris* L.) and pea (*Pisum sativum* L.), based on world production estimates. Chikpea is generally consumed as a seed food, being a good source of protein and other essential human nutrients. However, young chickpea leaves are also eaten as a cooked vegetable green in certain parts of the world and could be a useful source of dietary nutrients, especially in malnourished populations (Ibrikci et al., 2003). Chickpea seed contains 13 to 33% protein, 40 to 55% carbohydrates, 4 to 10% oil and fatty acids (50% oleic and 40% linoleic) (Berrada et al., 1999).

Nutraceutical Properties of Chickpeas

Kan et al., (2009) evaluated the antiviral activities of the extracts from the seed, fruit skin and aerial parts of ten registered varieties of *Cicer arietinum* (Chickpea) against *Herpes simplex* type 1 (*HSV*-1) and *Parainfluenza-3* (*PI*-3) viruses. Seed extracts of Cse-5 demonstrated good antiviral activity against both DNA (*HSV*-1; 32 - 4 μg ml-1) and RNA (*PI*-3; 32 - 16 μg ml-1) viruses compared among the seed (Cse), fruit skin (Cfs) and aerial part (Cap) extracts as well as the controls. Other seed extracts (Cse-4, Cse-7, and Cse-10) exerted selective inhibition against HSV at concentrations ranges of 32-16 μg ml-1, and 8-2 μg ml-1, respectively. Three fruit skin extracts (Cfs-3, Cfs-4, Cfs-9) were active against both *HSV*-1 and *PI*-3. Given, maximum non-toxic concentration, the remarkable antiviral activities were observed against HSV, in Cfs-4 (32 - 1 μg ml-1), Cfs-3 (32 - 8 μg ml-1), and Cfs-9 (32 -

4 μg ml-1), respectively. On the other hand, the activities against PI-3 were similar for Cfs-4 and Cfs-9 (32-16 μg ml-1), but different for Cfs-3 (32 - 4 μg ml-1). Cfs-6 and Cfs-7 had selective antiviral activity against *HSV*-1 at (32 - 16 μg ml-1), (32 - 2μg ml-1), respectively. This effect was observed for aerial part (Cap) extracts; as Cap-2, 4 (32 - 16 μg ml-1), Cap-5 (32 - 1 μg ml-1), and Cap-9 (16 - 2 μg ml-1). Only one (Cap-6) was active against both *HSV*-1 and *PI*-3. Cap-1 and 8 were selectively active against *PI*-3 at concentrations ranges of 16 - 8 and 32 - 8 μg ml-1, respectively.

Chickpeas contain daidzein, genistein, and formononetin (0.04, 0.06, and 0.14 mg/100 g, respectively), and approximately 1.7 mg/ 100 g biochanin A (Campos-Vega et al., 2010). Daidzein has garnered interest as a nontoxic compound capable of inducing tumor cell death in a variety of cancer types (Guo et al., 2004a; 2004b; Gercel-Taylor et al., 2004). Choi et al. (2008) showed that daidzein causes cell cycle arrest at the G1 and G2/M phases in human breast cancer cells. They also showed that while caspase-9 activity was significantly increased by daidzein, cyclin D expression decreased. *In vivo*, 9,10-dimethyl-1,2-dibenzanthracene-induced mammary tumors in rats were notably inhibited by daidzein and tumor latency was significantly increased in mouse mammary tumor virus-neu mice (Constantinou et al., 2001; Jin et al., 2002). Moreover, Ju et al. (2006) revealed that daidzein-induced MCF-7 cell proliferation was blocked by treatment with antiestrogen antibody Faslodex (ICI 182780), demonstrating that daidzein-induced stimulatory effect was estrogen receptor (ER) mediated. Jin et al., (2010) demonstrated that daidzein-induced apoptosis in MCF-7 cells is initiated by the generation of reactive oxygen species (ROS). Furthermore, daidzein-induced ROS generation accompanied by disruption of mitochondrial transmembrane potential, down-regulation of bcl-2, and up-regulation of bax, led to the release of cytochrome C from the mitochondria into the cytosol, which, in turn, result in the activation of caspase-9 and caspase-7, and ultimately in cell death.. The induction of the mitochondrial caspase-dependent pathway was confirmed by pretreatment with pan-caspase inhibitor z-VAD-fmk and antioxidant *N*-acetyl-L-cysteine (Figure 9).

Genistein (4′ ,5,7-trihydroxyisoflavone), the predominant isoflavone in human nutrition, is derived mainly from soybeans but also from other legumes like lentils (Perabo et al., 2008). *In vitro* studies have demonstrated that this natural compound downregulates the androgen receptor of PCa cells via the estrogen receptor *β*, resulting in a modified response to hormonal stimuli, inhibits several steroid-metabolizing enzymes such as 5-*α*-reductase or aromatase creating a more favorable hormonal milieu and a protective effect against prostate cancer, blocks the cell cycle progression at G1, and inhibits PSA expression (Perabo et al., 2008). With regard to its antioxidant activity, a study examined the effect of genistein on human prostate cancer (LNCaP and PC-3) cells. cDNA microarray analysis was performed to obtain the gene expression profile of genistein in LNCaP cells. This survey showed that while the expression of many genes, including apoptosis inhibitor (survivin), DNA topoisomerase II, cell division cycle 6 (CDC6), and mitogen activated protein kinase 6 (MAPK 6), was downregulated, the glutathione peroxidase (GPx)-1 gene expression level was upregulated with subsequent increase of GPx enzyme activities (Suzuki et al., 2002). Another interesting study investigated the potential additive and synergistic effects of genistein and resveratrol for suppressing prostate cancer in the Simian Virus-40 Tantigen (SV-40 Tag) targeted probasin promoter rat model, a transgenic model of spontaneously developing prostate cancer. High dose genistein and resveratrol treatments reduced cell proliferation and increased apoptosis mainly through the modulation of sex steroid receptor and growth factor signaling, suppressing the most severe grade of prostate cancer in these transgenic animals (Harper et al., 2009). In a randomized, placebo-controlled, double-blind phase II clinical trial, fifty-four study subjects were recruited and randomized to treatment with 30 mg genistein (n = 23) or placebo (n = 24) for 3 to 6 wks prior to prostatectomy. Serum prostate specific antigen (PSA) decreased by 7.8% in the genistein arm and increased by 4.4% in the placebo arm, without adverse events and with beneficial effect on blood cholesterol (Lazarevic et al., 2011).

A.

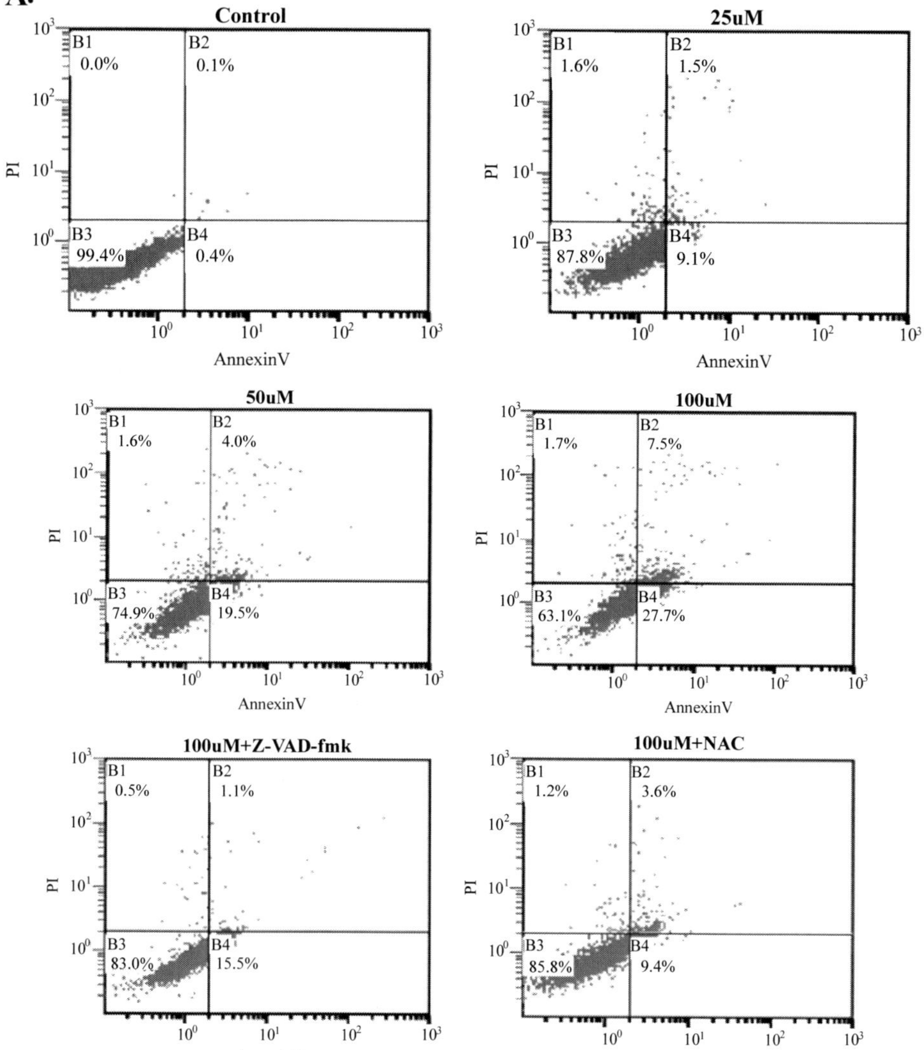

Figure 9. Daidzein induces apoptosis in MCF-7 cells. Representative flow cytometric analysis of MCF-7 apoptotic cells stained for Annexin V +propidium iodide (PI) after treatment with 0–100 μM daidzein, 100 μM daidzein + pan-caspase inhibitor z-VAD-fmk (100 μM), or antioxidant N-acetyl-Lcysteine (5 mM) for 24 h. In each panel, the lower right quadrant contains apoptotic cells (positive for Annexin V and negative for PI) (From Jin et al., 2010).

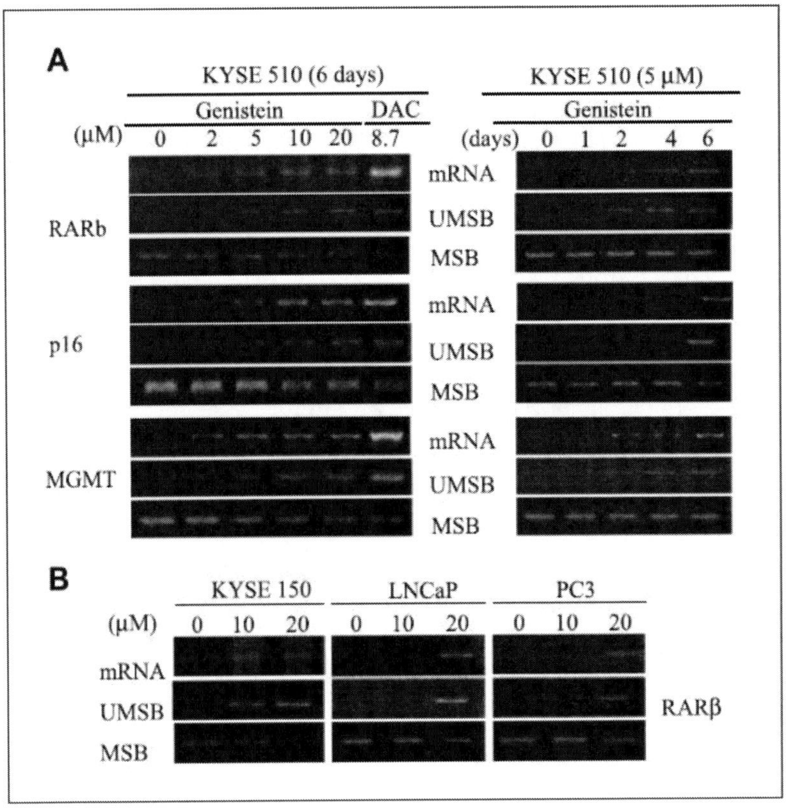

Figure 10. Alterations of methylation status and mRNA expression levels of RARb, p16, and MGMT genes after genistein treatment. Methylation status and mRNA expression level were determined with methylation-specific PCR and RT-PCR, respectively. UMSB, unmethylation-specific band; MSB, methylation-specific band. A, dose- and time-dependent alterations of methylation status and mRNA expression levels. Left, KYSE 510 cells treated with 2, 5,10, or 20 μmol/L of genistein or 8.7 μmol/L of 5-aza-dCyd (DAC) for 6 days. Right, cells treated for1, 2, 4, and 6 days with 5 μmol/L of genistein. B, alterations of methylation status and mRNA expression level of RARb gene in KYSE150, LNCaP, and PC3 cells. Cells treated with10 or 20 μmol/L of genistein for 6 days (From Fang et al., 2005).

Genistein (2-20 μmol/L) reverses DNA hypermethylation and reactivates *RARβ*, $p16^{INK4a}$, and *MGMT* in KYSE 510 cells (Figure 10). These effects by genistein are also observed in KYSE 150 cells and prostate cancer LNCaP and PC3 cells. Genistein (20-50 μmol/L) dose-dependently inhibited DNA methyltransferase activity, showing substrate- and methyl donor–dependent inhibition. Biochanin A and daidzein are less effective in inhibiting DNA methyltransferase activity, in reactivating *RARβ*, and in inhibiting cancer cell growth. In combination with trichostatin, sulforaphane, or 5-aza-dCyd, genistein enhances reactivation of these genes and inhibition of cell growth (Fang et al., 2005).

More recently, Bosviel et al., (2012) suggested that the treatment with 18.5 μM genistein or 78.5 μM daidzein might reverse DNA hypermethylation and restore the expression of the oncosuppressor genes BRCA1 and BRCA2 (Breast cancer 1 and 2, respectively). While 5-azacitydine (a demethylation agent) enhanced the reexpression of these genes, budesonide (a methylant agent) had an opposite effect. These observations, while requiring replication, provide new evidence on potential epigenetic mechanisms by which genistein and daidzein might contribute to regulation of the BRCA1 and BRCA2. Future studies are warranted on whether the demethylating effect of genistein and daidzein is global or focused on select candidate genes.

The molecular mechanisms involved in the effect of formononetin on prostate cancer cells has been studied by Ye et al., (2012), suggesting that higher concentrations of formononetin inhibit the proliferation of prostate cancer cells (LNCaP and PC-3), while the most striking effect was observed in LNCaP cells. Formononetin suppressed extracellular signal-regulated kinase1/2 (ERK1/2) mitogen-activated protein kinase (MAPK) signaling pathway in a dose-dependent manner, resulting in increased expression of Bcl2-associated (B-cell lymphoma 2) X (Bax) mRNA and protein, and induced apoptosis in LNCaP cells (Ye et al., 2012). This research concluded that the induced apoptosis effect of formononetin on human prostate cancer cells was related to ERK1/2 MAPK-Bax pathway. Formononetin also accelerate wound closure rate as early as 3 days after surgery and consistently observed until 10 days after in wound animal model. Huh et al., (2011) investigated the influence of formononetin on the expression of early growth response factor-1 (Egr-1) and growth factors contributing to wound healing. Formononetin significantly increased growth factors such as transforming growth factor-beta 1 (TGF-β1), vascular endothelial growth factor (VEGF), platelet-derived growth factor (PDGF) and basic fibroblast growth factor (bFGF) in human umbilical vein endothelial cells (HUVECs). Formononetin also increased the expression of Egr-1 transcription factor by 3.2- and 10.5-fold, compared with recombinant $VEGF_{125}$ in HUVECs. Western blot analysis of scratch-wounded confluent HUVECs showed that formononetin induced the phosphorylation of extracellular ERK and slightly inhibited the phosphorylation of p38 MAPK. The formononetin -mediated sustained activation of Egr-1 was suppressed by the ERK inhibitor PD98059 and the p38 inhibitor SB203580. These data suggest that formononetin promotes endothelial repair and wound healing in a process involving the over-expression of Egr-1 transcription factor through the regulation of the ERK1/2 and p38 MAPK pathways.

Manna (2012) found that biochanin, a methoxy form of genistein, inhibits IL-8-mediated activation of nuclear transcription factor kappaB (NF-κB) and activator protein 1 (AP-1) more potently than genistein in Jurkat T-cell line. Both biochanin and genistein potently inhibited nonreceptor protein-tyrosine kinases Lck and Syk activity, but biochanin specifically inhibited IKK activity. Biochanin completely inhibited NF-κB activation induced by peroneal muscular atrophy (PMA), lipopolysaccharide, pervanadate (PV), or H_2O_2, but only partially induced by TNFα. (tumor necrosis factor). Genistein was unable to inhibit IL-8-induced (interleucine-8) IKK (IkappaB kinase) activity, but it blocked PV-induced IKK activity. Biochanin completely inhibited NF-κB activation by TRAF6, but partially by TRAF2 (TNF receptor associated factors 6 and 2, respectively). *In silico* data suggested that biochanin interacted strongly with serine/threonine kinase than genistein, though both equally interacted with PTK. The data showed that both biochanin and genistein are potent inhibitors of PTK, but biochanin is a potent inhibitor of serine/threonine kinase too. Formononetin, having hydroxyl methoxy group is less potent to inhibit IKK than biochanin. Biochanin inhibits NF-κB activation not only by blocking the upstream IKK, but also PTK that phosphorylate tyrosine residues of IκBα. Thus, the double-edged sword effect of inhibition of NF-κB *via* inhibition of both serine/threonine kinase and PTK by biochanin might show useful therapeutic value against activities of cells that lead to tumorigenesis and inflammation. Similar results were observed by Kole et al., (2011); their investigation demonstrated that,

Biochanin-A inhibited lipopolysacharide (LPS)-induced nitric oxide (NO) production in macrophage and dose dependently inhibited inducible nitric oxide synthase (iNOS) expression. The induction of NF-κB binding activity by LPS was inhibited markedly by co-incubation with different doses of Biochanin-A. Biochanin-A inhibited the LPS-induced IKK activity and NF-κB activation associated with the inhibition of iNOS expression. LPS-induced phosphorylation of IκBα and p38 MAPK was blocked by Biochanin-A and it inhibited IL-6, IL-1β and TNF-α production in RAW264.7 cells demonstrating its anti-inflammatory activity in association with anti-proliferation.

Most plant-derived foods contain low to moderate levels of vitamin E activity. However, owing to the abundance of plant-derived foods in our diets, they provide a significant and consistent source of vitamin E. Tocopherol content is higher in grains and legumes than cereals. Chickpeas contain similar levels of α- and β + γ-tocopherols (6.9 and 5.5 mg/100 g, respectively) (Campos-Vega et al., 2010). Pregnant ewes were individually given daily oral supplements of 500 mg of alpha- tocopherols (aT), 1000 mg of gamma- tocopherols (gT), or placebo (CON) from 107 to 137 d post breeding to determine their effects on serum concentrations of 8-epi-prostaglandin F2 alpha (isoprostane) and adiponectin, mRNA expression of peroxisome proliferator-activated receptor gamma (PPARγ), adiponectin (ADIPQ), and related genes in the uterus and placentome (Kasimanickam and Kasimanickam, 2011). The mRNA abundance for PPARγ in the cotyledon and caruncle were similar in aT and gT ewes. The PPARγ, ADIPQ and LEP mRNA expressions were reduced ($P < 0.05$) in the cotyledon and caruncle in aT versus CON ewes. However, PPARγ mRNA expression with ADIPQ and LEP mRNA expressions were inversely associated in cotyledons, positively related in the caruncle, and positively downregulated in the uterus in gT supplemented ewes accounting for CON. The IGF-1 mRNA expression was downregulated in the cotyledon, caruncle and uterus in aT supplemented ewes. Expression of IGF-2 mRNA was upregulated in the cotyledon and caruncle, and downregulated in the uterus in gT supplemented ewes. Oral supplementation of tocopherol during late gestation in ewes decreased isoprostane concentrations and increased adiponectin concentrations in the serum, and significantly affected PPARγ- and ADIPQ-related genes in the utero-placental network. An original article published by Ahn et al., (2011) informed that vitamin E had a positive effect on gene expressions regarding osteogenic differentiation of mesenchymal stem cells. It was found that vitamin E enhanced cell proliferation when compared to cells cultured in media without vitamin E. They focused on 68 genes related to osteogenesis and osteoclastogenesis. Alkaline phosphatase, transforming growth factor-beta 1 (TGF-beta1), fibroblast growth factor receptor 1 (FGFR-1), matrix metalloproteinase 2 (MMP-2), muscle segment homeobox 2 (Msx-1), bone morphogenetic protein 1 (BMP-1), biglycan, vascular endothelial growth factor B (VEGF-B), dentin sialophosphoprotein (Dspp), cartilage oligomeric matrix protein (COMP), runt-related transcription factor 2 (RUNX-2), fibroblast growth factor receptor 3 (fgfr3), and SMAD2 were upregulated > 2-fold compared to the control. Conversely, osteopetrosis-associated transmembrane protein 1, microphthalmia-associated transcription factor, and epidermal growth factor receptor were downregulated > 2-fold compared to the control. Vitamin E produced a 1.5-fold increase in the expression of runt-related transcription factor 2 and transforming growth factor-beta 1 as determined by real time RT-PCR (Ahn et al., 2011).

Phytic acid (PA; myo-inositol hexaphosphate or $InsP_6$), a major phosphorus storage form in plants, and its salts known as phytates regulate various cellular functions such as DNA repair, chromatin remodeling, endocytosis, nuclear messenger RNA export and potentially hormone signaling important for plant and seed development (Zhou and Erdman, 1995), as well as animal and human nutrition (Vucenik and Shamsuddin, 2006). $InsP_6$ – the most abundant inositol phosphate in dry legumes is considered the anticancer agent. The most abundant inositol phosphate in raw, dry legumes is $InsP_6$, accounting for an average of 83% of the total inositol phosphates, ranging from 77% in chickpeas.

PA affects the cell cycle by decreasing the S-phase of mitosis and arresting cells in the G0/G1 phase. Shamsuddin and Ullah (1989) reported that PA significantly lowered the mitosis rate in AOM-induced colon tumors in Fisher 344 rats. PA also up-regulates expression of the tumor suppressor genes *p53 and p21 waf1/Cip1* (Saied and Shamsuddin 1998). Xu et al., (2011) suggested that IP6 protects against 6-hydroxydopamine -induced cell apoptosis in both normal and iron-excess conditions, and may offer neuroprotection in Parkinson's disease. Anekonda et al., (2011) identified potential novel functions of PA—a moderate up-regulation of SIRT1 (sirtuin 1), PAMPK (Phosphorylated AMP kinase)/AMPK ratio, and autophagy proteins. They proposed a potential mechanism of protection by PA in mouse brain.

PA attenuates oxidative stress, which in turn may lead to increased SIRT1 function and an increased PAMPK/AMPK. This results in improved autophagy and mitochondrial functions. These events together may have multiple complementary effects in reducing AP180 expression, Aβ production, attenuation of intracellular calcium increases, and overall plaque pathology in PA-treated animals.

PA also has an inhibitory effect on HepG2 cell proliferation (human hepatoma cell) and its mechanism might be related to many factors, such as inhibiting the abnormal expressions of cyclinD1 and CDK4 (Cyclin-dependent kinase 4), and inducing the expressions of cell cycle inhibitor Rb (retinoblastoma) and p27 (Xin and Yang, 2011).

Additionally, IP6 can suppress the proliferation and induce apoptosis of HT-29 cells. Longer IP6 treatment induced stronger apoptosis. Caspase3 plays an important role in the regulatory mechanisms of cell apoptosis as confirmed by RT-PCR assay (Li and Yang, 2008). Kapral et al., (2012) informed that IP6 exerts its anti-metastatic activity through modulation of MMP (Matrix metalloproteinases) and TIMP (Tissue Inhibitor of Metalloproteinases) genes expression to prevent cancer cell migration and invasion. Agarwal et al., (2004) revealed the anticancer efficacy of IP6 against hormone-dependent human prostate carcinoma PCA LNCaP cells, which involves inhibition of cell cycle progression in G1 phase and apoptotic induction. IP6 upregulates CDKIs accompanied by its increased binding with cyclin-dependent kinases (CDKs), causing a strong reduction in their kinase activity (Figure 10).

This leads to further decrease in the hyperphosphorylated form of Rb (ppRb) with a concomitant increase in its hypophosphorylated form, increasing binding of transcription factors E2Fs with pRb in the cytoplasm, thereby reducing their transcriptional activity for growth-responsive genes. This effect is also augmented by a decrease in some E2F levels by IP6. Furthermore, IP6 inhibits Akt activation and showed an overall increase in Bax/Bcl2 ratio, which might be prominent mechanisms for the apoptotic death of PCA cells (Figure 11).

An interesting study was carried out to seek the molecular mechanism of inositol hexaphosphate (InsP6) action that may inhibit proliferation of colon cancer cells and cell cycle progression (Węglarz et al., 2006).

A kinetic study of *p53* and *p21WAF1* mRNA increase was performed on human colon cancer HT-29 cells after treatment with 1, 5 and 10 mM InsP6 for 6, 12, 24 and 48 h. InsP6 stimulated *p53* and *p21WAF1* expression at the mRNA level, with the highest increase in *p21WAF1* mRNA occurring at 24 h, i.e., following the highest increase in *p53* mRNA observed at 12 h. The ability of InsP6 to arrest the cell cycle may be mediated by the transcriptional up-regulation of the p53-responsive *p21WAF1* gene (Figure 12).

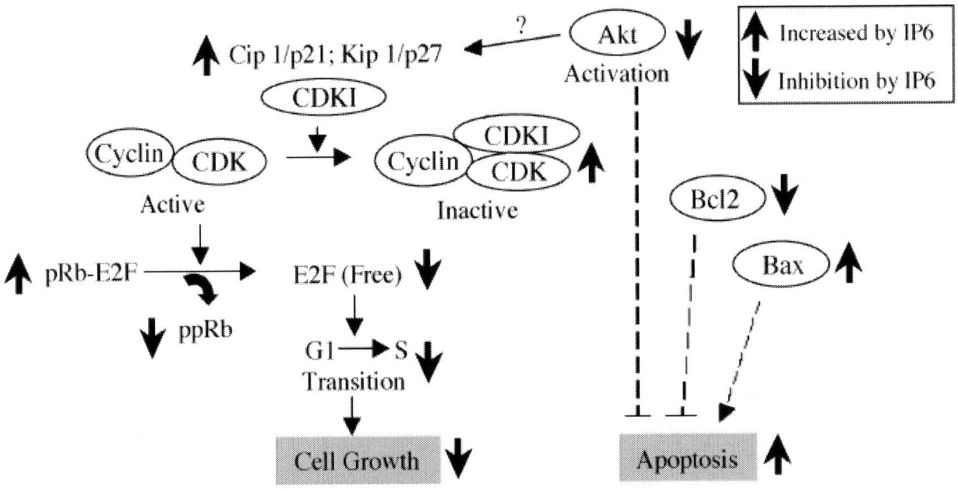

Figure 11. Proposed mechanisms of anticancer efficacy of IP6 associated with G1 arrest in cell cycle progression and apoptosis induction in human prostate carcinoma LNCaP cells (From Agarwal et al., 2004).

Saponins are a chemically heterogeneous group of steroid and triterpenoid glycosides present in a wide range of plant species. The saponin dehydrosoyasaponin I is a natural product present in chickpeas and other legumes and known as a potent calcium-activated potassium channel opener and as such can be used for treating cardiovascular, urological, respiratory, neurological, and other disorders (Taylor and Richards, 2008). Sialylation involving tumor formation and invasive behavior goes along with altered sialyltransferase (ST) activity.

SoyasaponinI (SsaI), a potent ST inhibitor, was discovered to selectively inhibit the cellular α2,3-sialyltranserase activity. Hsu et al., (2005) further tested the effects of SsaI on modifying the metastatic and invasive behaviors of cancer cell lines. SsaI successfully inhibited cellular α2,3-ST activity and depressed the dose dependent tumor cell surface α2,3 sialic acid expression. In addition, different concentrations of SsaI stimulated MCF-7 cell adhesion to collagen type I linearly and significantly enhanced cell adhesion to the Matrigel-matrix.

Furthermore, SsaI significantly decreased MDA-MB-231 (breast cancer) cell migration. Reverse transcriptase polymerase chain reaction for evaluating mRNA expression of ST3Gal I, III and IV showed that SsaI also down-regulated the expression of ST3Gal IV, but did not affect the other two.

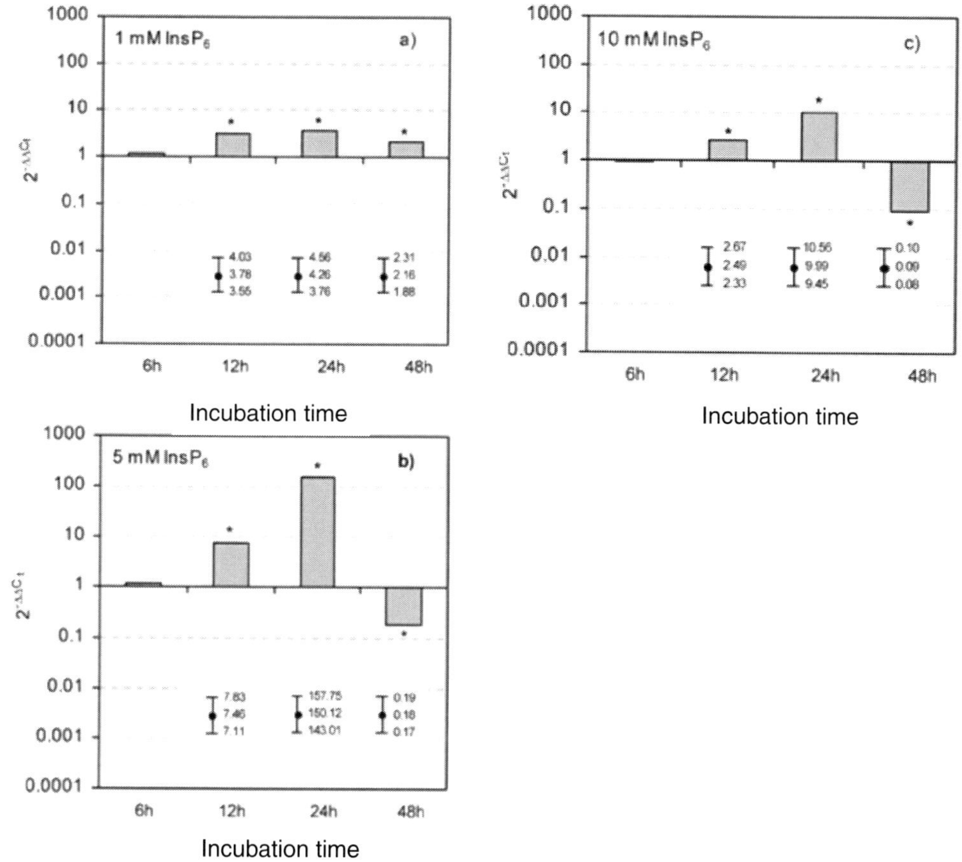

Figure 12. Changes in *p21WAF1* mRNA expression in HT-29 cells after treatment with InsP6 for 6, 12, 24 and 48 h compared to control cells. Detection and quantification of *p21WAF1* mRNA in total cellular RNA was performed by RT-PCR and ABI PRISM Sequence Detection System. The value of 2–ΔΔCt represents the expression of the *p21WAF1* gene in InsP6-treated cells normalized to β-actin relative to the normalized expression of *p21WAF1* gene in control cells. Mean values of ΔΔCt and error range are also shown. $^*P < 0.05$ *vs* control cells (Adapted from Węglarz et al., 2006).

Chickpeas as a functional food ingredient may be beneficial for correcting dyslipidaemia and preventing diabetes. The improved effects of dietary chickpeas on visceral adiposity, dyslipidaemia and insulin resistance were examined by Yang et al., (2007). Rats were fed a normal-fat diet (NFD), a high-fat diet (HFD) or a high-fat plus chickpea diet (HFD+CP) for 8 months. The activities of lipoprotein lipase (LPL) in epididymal adipose tissue and hepatic TAG lipase in liver increased by 40 and 23 %, respectively in HFD rats compared with those in NFD rats; dietary chickpeas completely normalised the levels. Furthermore, chickpea-treated obese rats also showed a markedly lower leptin and LPL mRNA content in epididymal adipose tissue. An insulin tolerance test, oral glucose tolerance test and insulin-releasing test showed that chickpeas significantly improved insulin resistance, and prevented postprandial hyperglycaemia and hyperinsulinaemia induced by the chronic HFD.

LENTILS

Of the Leguminoceae family, lentils (*Lens culinaris* L) are nowadays considered among the most important legumes for human nutrition (Iqbal et al., 2006). A variety of lentils exists with colours that range from yellow to red-orange to green, brown and black. Lentils are divided into two main types based on difference between the seed coat and cotyledon colour. Green lentils (Macrosperma) have a green to brown seed coat with yellow cotyledons. Red lentils (Microsperma) have a pale grey to dark seed coat with red cotyledons. Like most legumes, lentil seeds contain about two-thirds carbohydrates, 24–30% protein and are also a good source of B-complex vitamins, such as folate, thiamine, niacin and riboflavin, with a good balance of minerals (Jood et al., 1998; Longnecker et al., 2002). Lentil seeds provide an excellent source of dietary fiber and complex carbohydrates (Sotomayor et al. 1999). Lentil seeds are rich sources of proteins (Iqbal et al., 2006) and bioactive peptides, including lectins (Cuadrado et al., 2002), "defensin" protein (Finkina et al., 2008), and Bowman-Birk trypsin inhibitors (Losso, 2008); each of which aids in halting tumorigenesis and has gained special attention for its inhibitory effect against colorectal cancer (Mejia et al., 2005; Clemente et al., 2005).

Nutraceutical Properties of Lentils

Flavonoids are group of polyphenolic compounds, known to have significant anti-tumor, antioxidant and anti-inflammatory activities (Hodek et al., 2002). The flavan-3-ol and flavone content of eleven lentil cultivars grown in the northern United States has been reported (Xu and Chang, 2010). Two major flavan-3-ols [(+)-catechin and (-)-epicatechin] and one flavone (luteolin) were detected with the flavan-3-ols as the major flavonoids in all lentil cultivars. The content of (+) – catechin and (-)-epicatechin ranged from 267 and 2535 μg/g in Crimson to 1899 and 4947 μg/g in Morton, respectively. Luteolin content ranged from 21.8 μg/g in CDC Richlea to 77.1 μg/g in French Green. Luteolin, 3',4',5,7-tetrahydroxyflavone exert immunomodulatory effects that may be beneficial in the treatment of neurodegenerative diseases such as multiple sclerosis (MS), which has an underlying T-cell mediated autoimmune pathology (Stadelmann, 2007). *In vitro* studies show that luteolin inhibits T cell activation (Chen et al., 2004) and reduces the proliferation of autoreactive T-cells induced by both alpha B-crystallin and the murine encephalitogen proteolipid protein peptide (PLP), candidate autoantigens in MS and experimental autoimmune encephalomyelitis (EAE), respectively (Verbeek et al., 2004). In addition, luteolin blocks myelin basic protein-induced mast cell's stimulation which is capable of activating T-cells (Theoharides et al., 2008; Kempuraj et al., 2008). Luteolin reduces the proliferation of peripheral blood mononuclear cells (PBMCs) dose-dependently, and modulate IL-1β and interferon-beta (IFN-β) levels released by PBMCs in the culture supernatants. Luteolin reduces the MMP-9/TIMP-1 ratio by lowering MMP-9 production. Generally, luteolin has additive effects in modulating cell proliferation, IL-1β, TNF-α, cell migration mediator MMP-9 and it´s inhibitor TIMP-1 when combined with IFN-β (Sternberg et al., 2009). Qiao et al., (2012) recently informed that luteolin protects the brain from damage caused by permanent middle cerebral artery occlusion, and this effect may be through downregulation of TLR4, TLR5 (toll-like receptor),

NF-κB, p38MAPK and upregulation of ERK expression. Additionaly, luteolin could inhibit the proliferation of A549 cells (lung adenocarcinoma cells) via induction of apoptosis, with the evidence of characteristic morphological changes of apoptosis in the nucleus. Furthermore, luteolin induces S phase arrest of the cell cycle. The membrane potential of mitochondria also decreases. The protein levels of Bax, Bcl-xl, Bcl-2, Mcl-1, caspase-9, caspase-3, and PARP (apoptosis related proteins) were activated after treatment with luteolin (Chen et al., 2012).

On the other hand, food extracts with a high (−)-epicatechin content exert systemic anti-inflammatory actions. Vazquez-Prieto et al., (2012) investigated the capacity of (−)-epicatechin to prevent tumor necrosis alpha (TNFα)-induced activation of cell signals involved in inflammation and insulin resistance (NF-κB, mitogen-activated protein kinases (MAPKs), AP-1, and peroxisome proliferator activated receptor γ (PPARγ)) in differentiated white adipocytes (3T3-L1). TNFα triggered the activation of transcription factors NF-κB and AP-1, and MAPKs ERK1/2, JNK, and p38. (−)-Epicatechin (0.5–10 μM) decreased TNFα-mediated JNK, ERK1/2, and p-38 phosphorylation, and nuclear AP-1-DNA binding dose-dependently. It also inhibited TNFα-triggered activation of the NF-κB signaling cascade, preventing TNFα-mediated p65 nuclear transport and nuclear NF-κB-DNA binding. (−)-Epicatechin also attenuated the TNFα-mediated downregulation of PPARγ expression and decreased nuclear DNA binding. Accordingly, (−)-epicatechin inhibited TNFα-mediated altered transcription of genes (MCP-1, interleukin-6, TNFα, resistin, and protein-tyrosine phosphatase 1B) involved in inflammation and insulin signaling. It can attenuate TNFα-mediated triggering of signaling cascades involved in inflammation and insulin resistance. Epicatechin provides gastroprotection by reinforcing the mucus barrier and neutralizing gastric juice and this protection occurs through the involvement of sulfhydryl compounds, α2-adrenoceptors, superoxide dismutase, nitric oxide, and heat shock protein-70 (Rozza et al., 2012). Epicatechin induces NF-κB, activator protein-1 (AP-1) and nuclear transcription factor erythroid 2p45-related factor-2 (Nrf2) via phosphatidylinositol-3-kinase/protein kinase B (PI3K/AKT) and extracellular regulated kinase (ERK) signalling in liver hepatocellular cells (HepG2) (Granados-Serrano et al., 2010).

On the other hand, a validated three-stage continuous fermentative system simulating the human colon was used to resemble the complexity and diversity of the intestinal microbiota and to investigate the impact of four flours (wholegrain rye, wholegrain wheat, chickpeas and lentils 50:50, and barley milled grains), characterized by naturally high dietary fiber content, on the intestinal microbiota composition and metabolomic output. All four flours showed positive modulations of the microbiota composition and metabolic activity confirmed by Fluorescence in situ hybridization and HT29 cell-growth curve assay (Maccaferri et al., 2012).

Phytosterols promote apoptosis (programmed cell death), an important mechanism in the inhibition of carcinogenesis, as illustrated by Woyengo et al., (2009) (Figure 13).

In pulses, phytosterols are present in small quantities, and the most common phytosterols are β-sitosterol, campesterol, and stigmasterol. Lentils contain good levels of tocopherol, sitosterol, campesterol, stigmasterol and squalene (4.5, 123.4, 15, 20 and 0.7 mg/100g, respectively) (Campos-Vega et al., 2010). β-sitosterol inhibits vascular smooth muscle cells proliferation by increasing the levels of p21cip1 protein, which in turn inhibits the CDK2 activity, and finally interrupts cell cycle progress (Chien et al., 2010). It also induces G_2/M arrest, endoreduplication, and apoptosis through the Bcl-2 and PI3K/Akt signaling pathways in human leukemia cells (U937 and HL60) (Moon et al., 2008). Jesch et al., (2009) tested the hypothesis that plant sterols can modulate the expression of transporters such as Niemann-Pick C1-like 1 (NPC1L1) and scavenger receptor class B, type I (SR-BI) to lower intestinal cholesterol absorption. FHs 74 Int cells, a human small intestine epithelial cell line, were treated with sitosterol, stigmasterol, and cholesterol. Sitosterol, but not stigmasterol, reduced the mRNA levels of NPC1L1 and HMG-CoA reductase similar to cholesterol. Sitosterol can inhibit the expression of NPC1L1 in the enterocytes, which could be an alternate mechanism for plant sterols to reduce intestinal cholesterol uptake. Sitosterol induces glucose uptake in adipocytes and stimulates adipogenesis in differentiating preadipocytes. Interestingly, although sitosterol displays general insulin-mimetic activity by stimulating glucose uptake and adipogenesis, it also induces lipolysis in adipocytes according to Chai et al., (2011). Furthermore, GLUT4 (glucose transporter) gene expression was highly down-regulated in sitosterol-treated adipocytes, compared to insulin-treated adipocytes, which was up-regulated. Insulin- and SIT-treated adipocytes showed similar levels of Akt, HSL (Hormone-sensitive lipase), and PI3 K (phosphoinositos 3-quinasa) gene suppression.

Table 1 Summarizes functional compounds present in pulses and their role on gene expression.

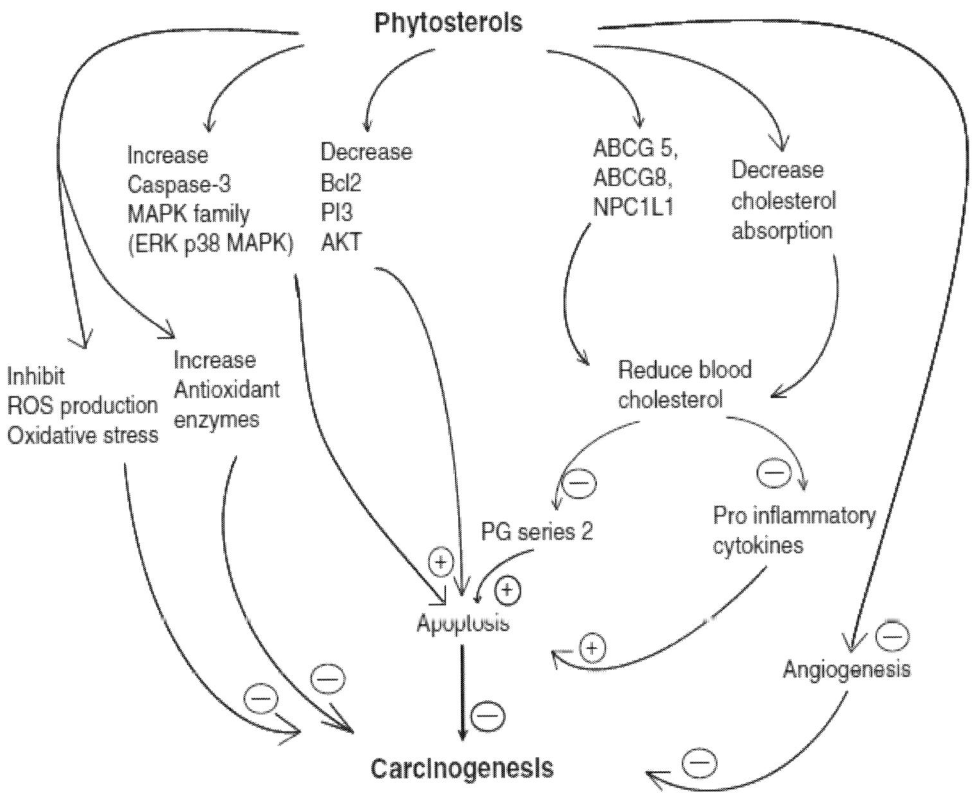

Figure 13. Proposed mechanism of action of phytosterols on carcinogenesis (From Woyengo et al., 2009).

Table 1. Role of pulse functional compounds on gene expression

Pulse-related compound	Modulated gene/action mechanism	Reference
Beans		
Fiber	*Hypocholesterolemic action* hepatic LDL receptor↑ SR-B1↑ cholesterol 7α-hydroxylase↑ hepatic HMG-CoA reductase↓	Han et al., (2004) Han et al., (2006)
Non-digestible fraction	*Colon cancer in vivo* β-catenin↓ p53↓ p21↑ Rb↓ Bax↑ Caspase-3↑	Feregrino-Pérez et al., (2008)
	Colon cancer in vivo Cell cycle arrest at the G1/S and G2/M phases, and apoptosis Tp53↑ Gadd45a↑ Cdkn1a↑ Bax↑ Cdc25c↓ Ccne2↓ E2f1↓ Bcl2↓ -DNA repair Xrcc4↑ Xrcc↑ PCNA↑	Vergara-Castañeda et al., (2012)
	Colon cancer in vitro -Cell cycle arrest at the G1 and G2/M phases SIAH1↑ p53↓ RB↓ p21↑ p16↑ Cyclin B2↑ Cdk1↓ Cyclin E2↓ -Apoptosis Bax↑ Bcl-2↑ Tnfrsf10b↑	Campos-Vega et al., (2010)
	Mamary carcinoma Bcl-2↓ X-linked inhibitor of apoptosis protein↓ Bax↑ Apoptosis protease-activating factor-1↑	Thompson et al., (2012)

Table 1. (Continued)

Pulse-related compound	Modulated gene/action mechanism	Reference
Phenolic compounds	*Mesenteric adipose tissue* TNF-α↓ MCP-1↓ IL-6↓	Kanamoto et al., (2011)
	Adipocytes PPARγ↑ C/EBPα↑ GLUT4↑ TNF-α↓ ROS↓	Inaguma et al., (2011)
	Aorta of spontaneously hypertensive rats NADPH oxidase subunits↓ iNOS↓ COX-2↓ MCP-1/CCR2↓	Mukai and Sato (2011)
	HeLa cells Bax↑ Caspase-3↑	Aparicio-Fernández et al., (2008)
Isoflavones	*Obesity* Genes involved in lipid metabolism, regulation of transcription and translation, protease inhibition, apoptosis, and cell proliferation	Iqbal et al., (2002)
	Estrogen-like activities Estrogen receptor in cytoplasm↑ progesterone receptor↑	Zhao et al., (2007)
Lectins	*Skeletal muscle in rats* GLUT-4↑ insulin receptor↑	Knott et al., (1992)
	Human breast cancer cells Fas↑ Caspase-8↑ Truncated BID↑ p53↑ Truncated Lamin A/C↑	Lam and Ng (2011)
Peas		
Proteins	*Hypolipidemic action in rats* SREBP-2↑ HMG-CoA↑ LDL receptor↑ CYP7A1↑	Spielmann et al., (2007)
	LDL receptor↑ SREBP-1c↓ FAS↓ SCD1↓ SCD2↓	Rigamonti et al., (2010)
	Spontaneously hypertensive rats - Anti-hypertension action Renin ↓	Li et al., (2011)

Pulse-related compound	Modulated gene/action mechanism	Reference
Carotenoids	*Colon cancer in vivo* Chaperones HSPD1↓ -Cell cycle p21↑ -Apoptosis Interleukin 18↑ *Lung cancer in vivo* HBA-A1↓ GSR↑ LDLR↑	van Breda et al., (2005a) van Breda et al., (2005b)
Phenolic compounds	Antioxidant capacity↑ Antioxidant activity↑ Antiradical activity↑	Xu et al., (2007) Amarowicz and Troszyñska (2003)
Chickpeas		
Daidzein	*Human breast cancer* -Cell cycle arrest at the G1 and G2/M phases Cyclin D↓ Caspase-9↓ -Apoptosis Bcl-2↓ Bax↑ Caspase-9↑ Caspase-7↑ -Reverse DNA hypermethylation BRCA1↑ BRCA2↑	Choi et al., (2008) Jin et al., (2010) Bosviel et al., (2012)
Genistein	*Breast cancer* -Reverse DNA hypermethylation BRCA1↑ BRCA2↑	Bosviel et al., (2012)
Formononetin	*Prostate cancer cells* - Proliferation inhibition ERK1/2/MAPK pathway↓ Bcl-2↑ *Human umbilical vein endothelial cells* -Endothelial reparation TGF-β1↑ VEGF↑ PDGF↑ bFGF↑ Egr-1↑	Ye et al., (2012) Huh et al., (2011)
Biochanin (methoxy form of genistein)	*Human T cell lymphoblast* -Inflamation/proliferation inhibition IL-8, IL-6, IL-1β↓ NF-κB↓ AP-1↓ Lck↓	Manna (2012)

Table 1. (Continued)

Pulse-related compound	**Modulated gene/action mechanism**	**Reference**
	Syk↓ IKK↓ PTK↓	
Vitamin E	*Osteogenesis and osteoclastogenesis* AP↑ TGF-beta 1↑ FGFR-1↑ MMP-2↑ Msx-1↑ BMP↑ Biglycan↑ VEGF-B↑ Dspp↑ COMP↑ RUNX-2↑ Fgfr3↑ SMAD2↑	Ahn et al., (2011)
Phytic acid (or $InsP_6$)	*Colon cancer* -G0/G1 cell cycle arrest and decreased S-phase of mitosis p21 wafl/Cip1↑ p53↑ *Improved autophagy* SIRT1↑ PAMPK/AMPK↑ *Human hepatoma cells* Cyclin D1↓ CDK4↓ Rb↑ P27↑ *Human prostate carcinoma* -Cell cycle G1 phase inhibition/apoptosis induction CDKIs↑ ppRB↓ E2F↓ Akt↓ Bax/Bcl2↑ Cip1/p21;Kip1/p27↑	Saied and Shamsuddin (1998); Węglarz et al., (2006) Anekonda et al., (2011) Xin and Yang, (2011) Agarwal et al., (2004)
Lentils	↑↓	
Luteolin		
	Proliferation of peripheral blood mononuclear cells MMP-9/TIMP-1↓	Sternberg et al., (2009)

Pulse-related compound	Modulated gene/action mechanism	Reference
	Brain protection from cerebral artery occlusion TLR4↓ TLR5↓ NF-κB↓ p38MAPK↓ ERK↓	Qiao et al., (2012)
	Lung adenocarcinoma -Apoptosis induction Bax↑ Bcl-xl↑ Bcl-2↑ Mcl-1↑ Caspase-9↑ Caspase-3↑ PARP↑	Chen et al., 2012
(−)-Epicatechin	*White adipocytes* -Inflammation and insulin resistance TNFα↓ JNK↓ ERK1/2↓ p-38↓ NF-κB↓ MCP-1↓ IL-6↓	Vazquez-Prieto et al., (2012)
β-Sitosterol	*Vascular smooth muscle* -Proliferation p21cip1↑ CDK2↑	(Chien et al., 2010)
	Leukemia -Apoptosis/Cell cycle arrest Bcl-2↑ PI3K/Akt↑	(Moon et al., 2008)
	Enterocytes -Intestinal cholesterol uptake reduction NPC1L1↓ HMG-CoA↓	Jesch et al., (2009)
	Adipocytes -Glucose update stimulation GLUT4↓	Chai et al., (2011).

TECHNOLOGICAL APPLICATIONS OF PULSES

At the turn of the 21st century, the industrialized world faces new challenges, that is, an enormous increase of health care costs, longer life expectancy, improved scientific knowledge, development of new technologies, and major changes in lifestyles. This has led to the idea of "optimal nutrition." Nutrition scientists want to rise to these new challenges and have embraced the idea of "optimal nutrition," which can be defined as the optimization of a daily nutrition model with nutrients and bioactive compounds to prevent diseases as well as to protect/maintain a healthy life. This approach has emerged due to increases in the costs of disease treatment, increased loss of work, and by consumer demand for a life with higher quality standards (Ashwell, 2002). The food industry can be a significant player in promoting wholesome diets, physical activity, and new product development in line with dietary guidelines. Initiatives have been undertaken by the food industry to reduce the levels of saturated fats, trans-fatty acids, sugars, and salt in processed foods, promote reasonable portion sizes, and increase the introduction of innovative, prudent, and nutritious choices. A review of current marketing practices could also accelerate health gains worldwide (WHO, 2008). Many in the food industry are increasingly turning to the power of pulses as a solution. Factors contributing to this include their reported nutritional and health benefits, changes in consumer preferences, increasing demand for variety/balance, changes in demographics (age, racial diversity), rise in the incidence of food allergies and ongoing research on production and processing technologies (Boye et al., 2010).

There is a wide range of opportunities to use pulses in the development of new products, including snacks, bakery, pastries, beverages, desserts, batter and breading, meat and meat analogues, soups and canned products. Pulse proteins are relatively low in methionine, cysteine and tryptophan but high in lysine and threonine, two essential amino acids. The introduction of legume flour into cereal products can therefore increase the protein, insoluble fiber, vitamin and mineral contents. Legumes and cereals are thus nutritionally complementary.

Production of canned pulses usually requires the following processing steps: blanching, soaking, canning and pasteurization. Canned baked beans, consisting of navy beans in tomato sauce, are one of the most popular bean products in the EU and USA (Mintel, 2005). Winham and Hutchins (2007) have shown that daily consumption of baked beans can reduce serum cholesterol in hypercholesterolemic adults.

Extrusion cooking has advantages including versatility, high productivity, low operating costs, energy efficiency and shorter cooking times. Legume extrusion has developed quickly in the last two decades. One of the benefits derived from pulse extrusion is enhancement of total dietary fiber (Berrios et al., 2010) or destruction of potentially antinutritional factors, especially protease inhibitors, hemagglutinins, tannins and phytates, which limit utilization of nutrients in legume seeds. Pulses, specially pea, chickpea and lentil, are rich sources of dietary fiber. Pulse fiber can be isolated by milling and fractionation of pulse seeds for incorporation into commercial food products to increase their fiber content and/or serve as functional ingredients (Meuser, 2001). Both hull fibres and cotyledon fibres made from peas are currently available for food applications. Commercially available pea fibres include the following: BCP Natural Pea Fiber (Best Cooking Pulses, Inc., Portage la Prairie, Canada); Uptake 80™, Accublend 50™, Centu-Tex™, and Century Flour™ (Nutri-Pea Ltd., Portage la Prairie, Canada); Exlite (Parrheim Foods, Saskatoon, Canada); Exafine® and Swelite® (Cosucra, Belgium); Pea Fiber IG (Roquette, France); and Vitacel® pea fibre (J. Rettenmaier, Germany) (Tosh and Yada, 2010). Berrios et al., (2010) reported an increase in dietary fiber content and a decrease in the concentration of the raffinose family of oligosaccharides upon extruding lentil, dry pea and chickpea flours.

Pulse extrusion also resulted in the development of a range of value added nutritious products such as pulse-based snacks or the fortification of cereal-based products such as pasta or tortilla with extruded pulse flours in order to enhance their amino acid profile. Extrusion cooking has also been applied in the production of instant type protein-rich porridge products by the incorporation of sorghum with cowpea as reported by Pelembe et al., (2002), who reported that addition of cowpea resulted in reduced viscosity of the developed instant porridge which could impact negatively on the acceptability of these products as food for adults. However, reduced viscosity could be very beneficial for infant feeding, and in addition, the nutritional impact could be of great importance, because sorghum has a low protein content and quality, particularly with respect to lysine, while cowpea rich in lysine, would complement the sorghum cereal and provide an opportunity for the production of a healthier extruded product.

Marzo et al., (2002) reported that the increase in all nutritional measurements in extruded kidney bean group compared with raw kidney bean showed that extrusion cooking is an effective treatment to reduce the toxicity of raw legumes. Extrusion cooking reduced phytic acid, condensed tannins, polyphenols, and trypsin, chymotrypsin, α-amylase inhibitory activity of the seeds, and hemagglutinating activity was completely eliminated. Body weight gain, protein efficiency ratio, and nitrogen concentration of sarcoplasmic and myofibrillar fractions also increased by methionine supplementation in an *in vivo* model, illustrating that kidney bean extrusion may be used to reduce the adverse impacts on performance and muscle metabolism caused by feeding raw beans. Alonso et al., (1998) demonstrated that the extrusion conditions: 148°C, 25% moisture and 100 rpm is effective in reducing condensed tannin, trypsin, chymotrypsin, α-amylase inhibitors and haemagglutinating activity in pea seeds, without modifying protein content as occurs by dehulling, soaking and germination treatments. In addition, trypsin and haemagglutinating activities in peas were more readily inhibited by extrusion treatment than chymotrypsin inhibitory activity.

Mora-Avilés et al., (2007) reported that protein content increased when nixtamalized maize flour of regular maize and commercial tortilla were combined with beans. The tryptophan and lysine as well as mineral contents in these tortillas increased. The maize and tortilla fortified with bean improved protein quality and could contribute significantly towards human nutrition, especially in countries like Mexico and Latin America where maize and beans are important components of the diet. Other study showed that tortillas fortified with different bean crops, had acceptable textural properties and significant improvement in their nutritional profile. Among the different crops studied, fortification with pinto bean flour showed great impact on the levels of phenolics and antioxidant activity, and a significant increase in crude protein levels (Anton et al., 2008). Cuevas-Martínez et al., (2010) demonstrated that up to 25% bean incorporation did not affect the physicochemical and textural properties of the tortillas. Consequently, as an alternative to solving the low protein quantity/quality of cereal-based foods problem caused by the their high starch content, 25% of added white bean increased lysine and tryptophan content in tortillas from 56 and 36% of FAO profile to 95 and 84%, respectively. In conclusion, the authors suggested the fortification of tortilla with white beans without modifications in the processing condition or equipment during tortilla production (Table 2).

The incorporation of legume flours with cereal flours for the extrusion of a new type of snack product with improved textural and nutritional characteristics has been extensively reported. The incorporation of navy and red bean flours with corn flour at 15, 30 and 45%

levels is one such attempt to produce fortified puffed snacks (Anton et al., 2009). In this study, the process variables of a twin screw extruder were kept constant (screw speed, moisture and temperature of the final zones at 150 rpm, 22% and 160 °C). Extrudates were produced using 30% bean flour with a level of crispness that was comparable to extrudates made from corn starch alone. At this level, crude protein increased 12- fold, and red bean fortification yielded extrudates with higher levels of phenols and both 2,2-diphenyl-1-picrylhydrazyl radical (DPPH.) and oxygen radical absorbance capacity (ORAC) compared to navy beans.

Table 2. Protein content and quality of raw grains and tortillas made with maize-bean blends

Component	FAO requirement	Raw grains Maize	Bean	Maize-bean ratios 100-0	95-5	90-10	85-15	80-20	75-25
Protein		94.80 ±1.17	210.40 ±6.64	91.53 ±0.29a	97.13 ±1.33b	100.53 ±0.46c	105.60 ±2.08d	110.27 ±0.92e	114.8 ±1.38f
Lysine	54.4	33.89 ±0.57	67.91 ±1.16	30.63 ±1.62a	36.98 ±0.25b	39.93 ±1.21c	43.33 ±0.65d	46.87 ±1.01e	51.84 ±0.46f
Tryptophan	9.6	7.28 ±0.11	32.90 ±1.89	3.45 ±0.27	4.26 ±0.09b	4.3 ±10.18b	5.67 ±0.07c	6.90 ±0.06d	8.04 ±0.01e

Mean of three replicates ± standard error. Mean values with same letter in the same row are not significantly different (Dunnet>0.05). Protein content in g/kg (dry basis). Amino acids are expressed in g/kg of protein (Adapted from Cuevas-Martínez et al., 2010).

The fortification of bakery goods with peas, beans and chickpea flours has already been employed and appears to be promising particularly for the functional food market (Dalgetty and Baik, 2006). The effect of utilizing pulse flours with coarse and fine particle size milled from green lentils (*Lens culinars*), yellow peas (*Pisum sativum* L.), navy beans (*Phaselous vulgaris* L.), and pinto beans (*Phaselous vulgaris* L.) was studied in pita bread and pan bread (Borsuk, 2011). Twenty five, 50, 75, and 100% pulse flours were used for pita baking, and 10, 15, and 25% for pan bread baking. Addition of pulse flours produced pitas with the pockets, but they were smaller in diameter and firmer in texture than the wheat control. Supplemented pan bread had lower specific loaf volume and firmer crumb with coarser grain. The recommended tolerance levels of pulse flour addition were 25% for pita bread and 10-15% for pan bread depending on the pulse flour and particle size. Navy and pinto beans were more suitable for baking applications. Cookies are another product that may be nutritionally improved through pulses addition. Cookies supplemented with roasted whole navy bean flour and high protein bean flour tend to have lower spread factors and breaking strengths than wheat flour cookies. On the other hand, bean-supplemented cookies have higher protein content and quality than wheat flour cookies (Dreher and Patek, 1984). Hoojjat and Zabik (1984) developed sugar-snap type cookies based on wheat flour supplemented with navy beans and sesame flours resulting in better baking properties and organoleptic characteristics than wheat flour cookies. Moreover, McWatters (1980) replaced milk protein with protein from cowpea and field pea flours in baking powder biscuits producing substantial changes in sensory quality attributes, crust and crumb colors, and density. The results open up a study area for product improvement, considering that the final product is also of high nutritional value. Tiwari et al., (2011) prepared biscuits by substituting wheat flour with dehulled pigeon pea (*Cajanus cajan* L) flour (PPDF) or pigeon pea byproduct flour (PPBF), which was obtained by recovering edible cotyledon material from milling byproducts. They obtained good quality biscuits with increased levels of protein and fibre using 85:15 of PPDF or 90:10 of PPBF without significantly affecting the sensory quality of biscuits. The study demonstrated the potential feasibility of incorporating pigeon pea milling byproducts in the manufacture of biscuits.

For the purpose of contributing to a healthy alternative for school snacks, Granito et al., (2010) recently developed three foodstuffs based on mixes of wheat and fermented and non-fermented legumes. They prepared cakes, brownies and cookies, where cakes were formulated substituting 20% of wheat flour with *Phaseolus vulgaris* flour, brownies with 30% of *Cajanus cajan* flour and cookies with 30% of *Vigna sinensis* flour, using fermented and non-fermented legumes in the three products. The sensory evaluation resulted in a high acceptability in the taste, color and overall appraised attributes for all the products, which was corroborated with a group of school children. Chemical characterization and calorie supply also resulted in an improvement of the products. They concluded that it is technically possible to incorporate fermented and non-fermented *Phaseolus vulgaris, Vigna sinensis and Cajanus cajan*, to highly consumed products such as cakes, brownies and cookies with a higher nutritional content and well-accepted by school-age children.

Pulse-fortified pasta offers consumers the possibility to improve the nutritional quality of their diet by offering enrichment in proteins and fibers, vitamins, minerals and amino acid complementarity. Petitot et al., (2010) suggested that pasta fortification with high levels of pulse flour presents a challenge and an opportunity to enhance the nutritional quality of a very popular food product and emphasized the optimization of the pastamaking process as the key to overcome sensory deficiencies when producing pulse-fortified pasta. Cabello et al., (1992) added 15% navy bean flour to microwavable pasta and like Bahnassey and Khan (1986) saw an improvement in nutritional value.

Zhao et al., (2005) developed spaghetti from semolina, containing 5% to 30% milled flours of green pea, yellow pea, chickpea, and lentil, respectively. The authors found that spaghetti containing legume flours darkened the spaghetti but did not affect the cooked weight significantly. Cooking loss and firmness increased with an increase in legume flour content. Moreover, the firmness, pulse flavor, and color intensity of the pasta products increased with increase in the percentages of legume flour fortification up to 30%, whereas the intensity of the shiny appearance, elasticity, and overall quality decreased. In addition, trypsin inhibitor activity (TIA/g) was significantly reduced after cooking. Finally, an important point when the product is finished, is to assess the acceptance by the consumer, and this study showed that consumers preferred control spaghetti (without legume additives) more than the spaghetti containing legume flours and they slightly liked the spaghetti with 15% lentil or green pea and the spaghetti with 20% chickpea or yellow pea. However, the introduction of legume-based products, which are relatively new to the population, could have a gradual acceptance over time, considering that it will finally improve the health of individuals.

Pulse starches have occupied an important place in noodle preparation in several countries of the world, and mung bean (*Vigna radiate*) has been reported as the best raw material for starch noodle preparation (Chen, 1978). Mung bean starch is favored for starch noodle production because it gives a product with the desired appearance and texture. The good quality achieved from mung bean starch is thought to result from the high amylose content and restricted granule swelling. The pasted starch exhibits a stable viscosity during heating and stirring test and a high setback on cooling (Lii and Chang, 1981). Noodles from navy and pinto bean starches have low quality compared to potato starch with respect to physicochemical properties, although navy and pinto bean starches have higher amylose contents than mung bean starch (Kim et al., 1996). Red bean starch noodles also have fairly good quality, although not as good as mung bean starch noodles (Lii and Chang, 1981). In contrast, Bourré (2012) found that addition of pulse flours (whole yellow peas, green lentils and navy beans) improved the nutritional profile of the noodles by increasing fibre and protein content.

The incorporation of pulse ingredients into meat products has also been a recent trend. Starch- and carbohydrate-rich fractions are often used as fat replacers in meat products and are good sources of slow-release carbohydrates. Pulse macromolecules can also interact with other components in the food matrix to create networks.

Adding pea ingredients to low-fat formulations decreases the percentage of water loss, indicating that the binders improve water retention in low-fat bologna sausages. Also, the addition of pea ingredients other than pea flour considerably improves the textural properties of the product, restoring the values of a low-fat product to levels equivalent to a regular-fat bologna (Pietrasik and Janz, 2010). Adding common bean flour to beef sausages results in lower shear force and hardness if a binder is not used (Dzudie et al., 2002).

Use of inner pea fiber in lower fat beef patties offers processors the opportunity of improved tenderness and cooking yield, without negative effects on juiciness and flavor. Inclusion of pea fiber in ground beef formulations may allow a lower fat beef patty to withstand prolonged heating while producing high cooking yields and acceptable eating quality. This may be desirable in food service facilities where longer cooking times are frequently employed to ensure microbial safety and lessen the presence of uncooked pink color (Anderson and Berry, 2000).

Modi et al., (2004) studied the effect of adding different decorticated legume flours, soya bean, bengal gram, green gram and black gram, on the quality of buffalo meat burger. The burgers prepared with any of these binders were organoleptically acceptable even after storage at −16°C for 4 months. The burger with black gram *dhal* (dehulled split legume) flour had better sensory quality attributes compared to other legumes.

For calorie-conscious people, a significant reduction in fat and total calories derived from fat can be achieved without affecting consumer acceptability in low-fat bologna, where pea and wheat flour can be combined for product development, because the fat is replaced with water and moisture content is directly proportional to the amount of added water (Pietrasik and Janz, 2010).

Some researchers have directed their studies towards using natural foods to fortify multipurpose beverages. Such is the case of legumes used recently in the beverage industry. A Mexican group research (Granito et al., 2004) developed a fermented dairy drink, partially substituted with clear varieties of *Phaseolus vulgaris* (caraota) and *Vigna sinensis* (frijol). The mixtures were inoculated with several bacteria (*Lactobacillus acidophillus, Streptococcus thermophilus and Bifidobacterium sp.*) using mango and guava jams as flavorings. Protein, soluble and insoluble fiber, available and resistant starch levels in the fermented dairy drinks increased and the protein digestibility was 81%. In conclusion, they authors suggested that the partial substitution of milk with extracts of *Phaseolus vulgaris* or *Vigna sinensis* may be a great option for the preparation of a fermented dairy drink similar to liquid yogurt.

Gluten intolerance or gluten sensitivity appears to have reached levels associated with other major health issues. Celiac disease is an auto-immune disorder triggered by gluten, a protein found in wheat, barley, rye and spelt. More than 20 million Americans may require gluten-free alternatives. For this reason, the demand to explore new alternatives to avoid gluten has increased in recent years. Advanced processing technology (heat and steam) is naturally producing precooked pulse flours with great functionality in gluten-free applications. In properly processed precooked flours the heat or steam partially gelatinizes the starch, denatures the protein, inactivates enzymes for longer shelf life, and, in general makes for a highly functional and versatile gluten-free mainstay. The slightly golden color and remarkably bland flavor of precooked yellow pea flour allows bakers to mimic the look and taste of the gluten-containing original products.

Han et al., (2010) reported the development of a gluten-free, 100% pulse-based cracker snack using pulse fractions including chickpea, green and red lentil, yellow pea, pinto and navy bean flours and pea proteins. The developed products scored highly during consumer acceptance testing; however, the beany flavor was found to be the greatest challenge to the development of successful pulse-containing crackers. In addition, while good crispness of crackers containing chickpea flour, red lentil flour and pinto flour was reported, the gluten-free nature of these products could inhibit the development of a texture resembling the wheatbased crackers familiar to many general consumers. Pea protein isolates are promising approach to produce protein enriched blends for making fermented gluten-free products (Marco and Rosell, 2008). Kinnikinnick Foods (Edmonton, Canada), a major producer of gluten-free foods uses pea fiber in many of their products (Tosh and Yada, 2010).

Addition of legumes to cereal products increases their content of fibre, resistant starch (Utrilla-Coello et al., 2007), important minerals (Dhingra and Jood, 2001; Dalgetty and Baik, 2003; Costa de Almeida et al., 2004) and vitamins. These products with addition of legumes have higher nutritive value compared to classical bread prepared from wheat or rye. Their consumption has positive impact on health conditions of consumers (Goni and Valentin-Gamazo, 2002; Johnson et al., 2005; Hawkins and Johnson, 2005; Pittaway et al., 2007). Apart from classical processing, legumes are also used to produce flour with specific granulation to be used in variety of food including pastries, bread, snacks, soups, mashed potatoes, etc. (Maaroufi et al., 2000).

A research was carried out to study characteristics of four gluten-free bread formulations and the possibility of substituting soya protein with other legume proteins (chickpea flour, pea isolate and carob germ flour) (Miñarro et al., 2012). Chickpea bread produced the softest crumb. Confocal scanning-laser microscopy results showed a more compact microstructure in carob germ flour bread compared with soya and chickpea formulations. Chickpea bread exhibited the best physico-chemical characteristics and, in general, good sensory behaviour, indicating that it could be a promising alternative to soya protein. Partial substitution of wheat flour with chickpea flour at 10, 20 and 30% levels affect bread quality in terms of volume, internal structure and texture (Mohammed et al., 2012). Experimental loaves prepared from mixtures of wheat flour and pulverized lentil and chickpea at 10 – 50 % showed lower volume, specific loaf volume, volume efficiency and cambering at higher level compared to control, according to Bojňanská et al. (2012). Nevertheless, from a nutritive standpoint the higher content of proteins with a suitable fraction structure and higher content of minerals with indispensable substances for humans are a significant contribution (Table 3). From the technological point of view chickpea appeared to be the most suitable raw material. Its addition at 10 % improved technological parameters of pastry. From the nutritive point of view, lentil is an excellent raw material. The best qualitative parameters (objective as well as subjective) are found in bread with addition of 10 % of chickpea.

Table 3. Nutritive quality of bread with chickpea and lentil

	Crumb acidity, Mmol/kg	Crude protein, %	Ash content, %
Control bread	45	12.57	0.80
Chickpea 10%	50	12.33	0.90
Chickpea 20%	56	12.99	1.10
Chickpea 30%	5	13.79	1.10
Chickpea 40%	61	14.70	1.30
Chickpea 50%	63	15.73	1.60
Control bread	30	10.53	1.11
Lentil 10%	33	12.50	1.38
Lentil 20%	40	13.13	1.44
Lentil 30%	50	14.43	1.75
Lentil 40%	60	15.49	1.82
Lentil 50%	76	16.28	2.13

From Bojňanská et al. (2012).

Chickpea addition at 20–40% in wheat cookies and 60–80% for amaranth and buckwheat cookies decrease the lightness in white wheat cookies while increasing it in whole wheat and amaranth cookies; it significantly increase yellowness in all cookies (Yamsaengsung et al., 2012). According to the authors, spread factor of the gluten-free cookies is reduced by chickpea addition and hardness is increased in white wheat and buckwheat cookies, and decreased in whole wheat and amaranth cookies. Sensory evaluation demonstrated that chickpea addition increased the acceptability of all cookies, particularly the gluten-free cookies. Also, extrusion technology has been used to develop acceptable snack products. Fenugreek in the form of deodorized powder (fenulife) could be incorporated up to 15% in a mixture of chickpea and rice to develop snack products of acceptable physical and sensory properties (Ravindran et al., 2007).

Gómez et al., (2008) informed that the addition of chickpea flour (50%) would improve the nutritional value of cakes without greatly affecting their quality characteristics. Lechoso and Sinaloa would be the most adequate cultivars for enrichment, and white better than whole flour. Sponge cake quality was less affected by the chickpea addition than layer cakes, probably because of the lower flour percentage in its formulation according to their results (Figure 14).

Blending various legumes with wheat flour, improves rheological and sensory characteristics of chapatti according to Shahzadi et al., (2005). The results also indicated that apart from the commercial flour, chapaties prepared from composite flour containing guar gum at 3%, 2% and chickpea 5%+ guar gum 1% level improved the sensory parameters of chapaties. However addition of lentil and chickpea at 10% could not make any significant impact on the sensory attributes. It was further observed that decrease in scores were almost linear to the percent replacement of lentil and chickpea.

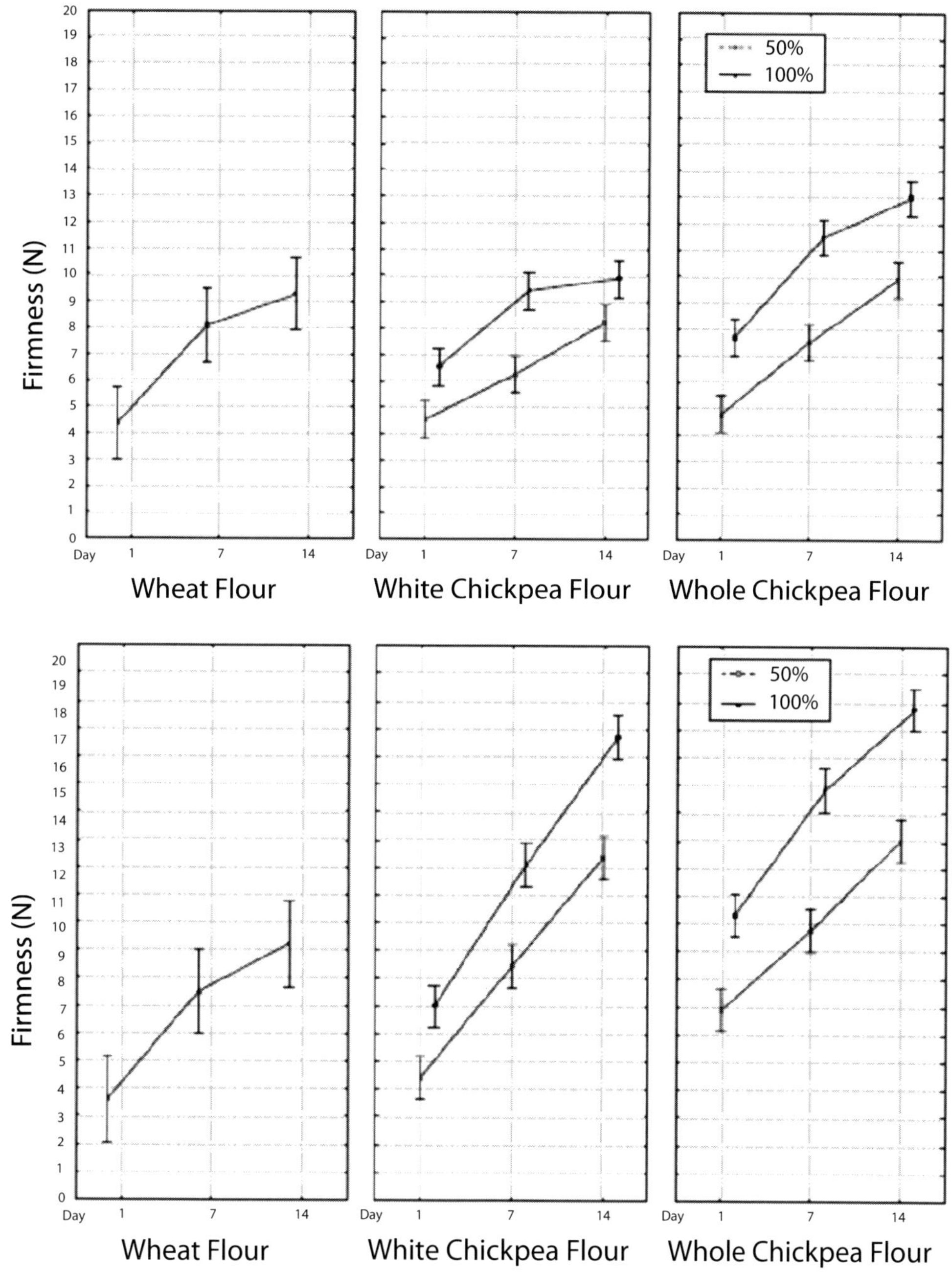

Figure 14. Effect of the composite flours on the firmness of cakes during storage obtained with 2 different recipes (Adapted from Gómez et al., 2008).

Chickpea yogurt fermentation hydrolyzes the isoflavone glucosides, and *L. bulgaricus* and *S. thermophilus* convert isoflavone glucosides to aglycones of daidzin and genistin (Fu et al., 2012). *L. bulgaricus* and *S. Thermophilus* seem to be effective starters for chickpea milk with more aglycones and appropriate acidity. As well, milk supplementation with pulse ingredients was examined as a means to increase the nutritional properties of yogurt and probiotic type beverages (Zare et al., 2012). The acid production rate of two yogurt starters (A and B) and two probiotic cultures (*Lactobacillus rhamnosus* and *Lactobacillus acidophilus*) was followed in milk supplemented with the following soy and pulse ingredients: pea protein, chickpea flour, lentil flour, pea fibre, soy protein concentrate and soy flour. All ingredients used for supplementation improved the acidification rate of probiotic cultures, and the highest effects were obtained with lentil and soy flour. The effect of ingredient supplementation on the microbial composition (ratio of cocci to bacilli) of the yogurt products was also examined. The ratio of cocci to bacilli was between 1.8 and 2.5 for all supplemented yogurt samples obtained with culture A, and these variations were not judged to be statistically significant ($p < 0.05$). With yogurt products obtained from culture B, however, there was a higher proportional level of lactobacilli in all supplemented samples, compared to the milk control; the enhanced growth of the lactobacilli was particularly noticeable when lentil flour was added to milk. Also, lentils enhance probiotic growth in yogurt and provide added benefit of antioxidant protection according to Agil et al., (2012). Results demonstrate that green lentils selectively enhance the number of probiotic bacteria in yogurt in the initial stages of storage and maintained overall microbial counts over a 28-day storage period. Adding lentil flour on layer and sponge cakes reduces layer cake volume and cohesiveness but increases hardness, and the total substitution gives harder cakes without tendency in volume (De la Hera et al., 2012).

Conclusion

Recent investigations suggest that pulses may contribute to human health and wellbeing, mostly through prevention of chronic diseases such as coronary heart disease, hypertension, cancer, diabetes and obesity. The interaction between nutrients present in pulses and gene modulation is emphasized. Advances in molecular biology have greatly contributed to a deeper understanding of the role of gene dietary modulation in disease prevention. Taking advance of the above, pulse food research trends reflect the emphasis of using pulses as ingredients in food product formulations. Regarding ingredient development, all pulses are being researched for their potential as ingredients in food products. More innovative pulse product development research currently underway includes the development of yogurts and pro-biotic products, gluten-free product formulations such as doughs and cookies among others.

References

Abou-Samra R, Keersmaekers L, Brienza D, Mukherjee R, Macé K. Effect of different protein sources on satiation and short-term satiety when consumed as a starter. *Nutr J.* 2011, 10:139.

Adamidou S, Nengas I, Grigorakis K,. Nikolopoulou D, Jauncey K. Chemical composition and antinutritional factors of field peas (*Pisum sativum*), chickpeas (*Cicer arietinum*), and faba bans (*Vicia faba*) as affected by extrusion preconditioning and drying temperatures. *Cereal Chem.* 2011, 88(1):80–86.

Adlercreutz H. Evolution, nutrition, intestinal microflora, and prevention of cancer: a hypothesis. *Proc Soc Exp Biol Med.* 1998, 217:241–246.

Agarwal C, Dhanalakshmi S, Singh RP, Agarwal R. Inositol hexaphosphate inhibits growth and induces G1 arrest and apoptotic death of androgen-dependent human prostate carcinoma LNCaP cells. *Neoplasia.* 2004, 6(5):646 – 659.

Agarwal S, Rao AV. Carotenoids and chronic diseases. *Drug Metab Drug Interact* 2000, 17(1–4):189–210.

Agil R, Gageta A, Gliwa J, Avis TJ, Willmore WG, Hosseinian F. Lentils enhance probiotic growth in yogurt and provide added benefit of antioxidant protection. *LWT - Food Sci Technology.* 2013, 50:45 - 49.

Ahn KH, Jung HK, Jung SE, Yi KW, Park HT, Shin JH, Kim YT, Hur JY, Kim SH, Kim T. Microarray analysis of gene expression during differentiation of human mesenchymal stem cells treated with vitamin E *in vitro* into osteoblasts. *Korean J Bone Metabol.* 2011, 18(1):23-32.

Alonso R, Orúe E, Marzo F. Effects of extrusion and conventional processing methods on protein and antinutritional factor contents in pea seeds. *Food Chem.* 1998, 63(4):505–512.

Alvarez Y, Briones AM, Hernanz R, Pérez-Girón JV, Alonso MJ, and Salaices M. Role of NADPH oxidase and iNOS in vasoconstrictor responses of vessels from hypertensive and normotensive rats. *Br J Pharmacol.* 2008, 153:926–35.

Amarowicz R, Pegg RB. Legumes as a source of natural antioxidants. *Eur J Lipid Sci Technol.* 2008, 110:865–878.

Amarowicz R, Troszyñska A. Antioxidant activity of extract of pea and its fractions of low molecular phenolics and tannins. *Pol J Food Nutr. Sci.* 2003, 12:10–15.

Amarowicz R. Tannins: the new natural antioxidants? *Eur J Lipid Sci Technol.* 2007, 109:549–551.

Anderson ET, Berry BW. Sensory, shear, and cooking properties of lower-fat beef patties made with inner pea fiber. *J Food Sci.* 2000, 65(5):805-810.

Anderson GH, Moore SE. Dietary proteins in the regulation of food intake and body weight in humans. *J Nutr.* 2004, 134:974S-979S.

Anderson JW, Johnstone BM, Cook-Newell M. Metaanalysis of the effects of soy protein intake on serum lipids. *New Engl J Med.* 1995, 333:276–282.

Anderson JW, Story L, Sieling B, Chen WJL, Petro MS, Story J. Hypocholesterolemic effects of oat-bran or bean intake for hypercholesterolemic men. *Am J Clin Nutr.* 1984, 40:1146–55.

Anderson JW. *Phytoestrogen effects in humans relative to risk for cardiovascular diseases, breast cancer, osteoporosis, and menopausal symptoms.* In: Pavlik EJ, ed. Estrogens, progestins, and their antagonists. Boston: Birkhauser, 1996:51–71.

Anekonda TS, Wadsworth TL, Sabin R, Frahler K, Harris C, Petriko B, Ralle M, Woltjer R, Quinn JF. Phytic acid as a potential treatment Phytic acid protects against 6-hydroxydopamine-induced dopaminergic neuron apoptosis in normal and iron excess conditions in a cell culture model for Alzheimer's pathology: evidence from animal and *in vitro* models. *J Alzheimers Dis.* 2011, 23(1):21-35.

Anton AA, Fulcher RG, Arntfield SD. Physical and nutritional impact of fortification of corn starch-based extruded snacks with common bean (*Phaseolus vulgaris* L.) flour: Effects of bean addition and extrusion cooking. *Food Chem.* 2009, 113(4):989–996.

Anton AA, Ross KA, Lukow OM, Fulcher RG, Arntfield SA. Influence of added bean flour (*Phaseolus vulgaris* L.) on some physical and nutritional properties of wheat flour tortillas. *Food Chem.* 2008, 109:33-41.

Aparicio-Fernández X, García-Gasca T, Yousef GG, Lila MA, González de Mejía E, Loarca-Piña G. Chemopreventive activity of polyphenolics from black Jamapa bean (*Phaseolus vulgaris* L.) on HeLa and HaCaT cells. *J Agric Food Chem.* 2006, 54:2116-2122.

Aparicio-Fernández X, Reynoso-Camacho R, Castaño-Tostado E, García-Gasca T, González de Mejía E, Guzmán-Maldonado SH, Elizondo G, Yousef GG, Lila MA, Loarca-Pina G. Antiradical capacity and induction of apoptosis on HeLa cells by a *Phaseolus vulgaris* extract. *Plant Foods Hum Nutr.* 2008, 63:35–40.

Aparicio-Fernández XO, Manzo-Bonilla L, Loarca-Piña GF. Comparison of antimutagenic activity of phenolic compounds in newly harvested and stored common beans *Phaseolus vulgaris* against aflatoxin B_1. *J Food Sci.* 2005, 70(1):73-78.

Ashwell M. 2002. *Concepts of functional foods.* Washington , D.C. : ILSI Europe Concise Monograph Series ILSI Press

Astrog P, Gradelet S, Berges R, Suschetet M. Dietary lycopene decreases initiation of liver preneoplastic foci by diethylnitrosamine in rat. *Nutr Cancer.* 1997, 29:60–68.

Auger C, Rouanet JM, Vanderlinde R, Bornet A, Decorde K, Lequeux N, Cristol JP, Teissedre PL. Polyphenols-enriched chardonnay white wine and sparkling pinot noir red wine identically prevent early atherosclerosis in hamsters. *J Agric Food Chem.* 2005, 53:9823–9.

Bahnassey Y, Khan K. Fortification of spaghetti with edible legumes. II. Rheological, processing and quality evaluation studies. *Cereal Chem.* 1986, 63:216-219.

Baird DD, Umbach DM, Lansdell L, Hughes CL, Setchell KD, Weinberg CR, Haney AF, Wilcox AJ, McLachlan JA. Dietary intervention study to assess estrogenicity of dietary soy among postmenopausal women. *J Clin Endocrinol Metab.* 1995, 80:1685–1690.

Barampama Z, Simard RE. Nutrient composition, protein quality and antinutritional factors of some varieties of dry beans (*Phaseolus Vulgaris*) grown in Burundi. *Food Chem.* 1993, 47:159-167.

Bazzano LA, He J, Ogden LG, Loria C, Vapputuri S, Myers L, and Whelton PK. Legume consumption and risk of coronary heart disease in US men and women. *Arch Intern Med.* 2001, 161(21):2573-2578.

Beninger CW, Hosfield GL. 2003. Antioxidant activity extracts, condensed tannin fractions, and pure flavonoids from *Phaseolus vulgaris* L. seed coat color genotypes. *J Agric Food Chem* 51:7879–83.

Berrada AM, Stack W, Riddell B, Brick MA, Johnson DL. Chickpea: A potential crop for southwestern Colorado. in *Perspectives on new crops and new uses.* Janick J. Ed., pp. 206-211, ASHS Press, Alexandria, VA 1999.

Berrios JJ, Morales P, Cámara M, Sánchez-Mata MC. Carbohydrate composition of raw and extruded pulse flours. *Food Res Int.* 2010, 43(2):531–536.

Bojňanská T, Frančáková H, Líšková M, Tokár M. Legumes- The alternative raw materials for bread production. *J Microbiol, Biotechnol Food Sci.* 2012, 1:876-886

Borsuk Y. Incorporation of pulse flours with coarse and fine particle size milled from green lentils (*Lens culinars*), yellow peas (*Pisum sativum* L.), navy beans (*Phaselous vulgaris* L.), and pinto beans (*Phaselous vulgaris* L.) into baked products. *FGS-Electronic Theses & Dissertations (Public).* 2011. http://hdl.handle.net/1993/4803.

Bosviel R, Dumollard E, Déchelotte P, Bignon YJ, Bernard-Gallon D. OMICS. *J Integr Biol.* 2012, 16(5): 235-244.

Bourdon I, Olson B, Backus R, Richter BD, Davis PA, Schneeman BO. Beans, as a source of dietary fiber, increase cholecystokinin and apolipoprotein B48 response to test meals in men. *J Nutr.* 2001, 131:1485–1490.

Bourré L. Incorporation of selected pulse flours into dried Asian white salted noodles. *FGS-Electronic Theses & Dissertations (Public).* 2012. URI: http://hdl.handle.net/1993/5225.

Boye J, Zare F, Pletch A. Pulse proteins: processing, characterization, functional properties and applications in food and feed. *Food Res Int.* 2010, 43:414–431.

Bunz F, Dutriaux A, Lengauer C, Waldman T, Zhou S, Brown JP, Sedivy JM, Kinzler KW, Vogelstein B. Requirement for p53 and p21 to sustain G2 arrest after DNA damage. Science. 1998, 282:1497-*1501.*

Burbano C, Muzquiz M, Ayet G, Cuadrado C, Pedrosa M. Evaluation of antinutritional factors of selected varieties of *Phaseolus vulgaris. J Sci Food Agric.* 1999, 79:1468–1472.

Cabello CS, Uebersax MA, Occena LG. Assessment of vean flour in conventionally cooked and microwave-prepared pasta. *Michigan Dry Bean Digest.* 1992, 16:7-9.

Cabrera C, Lloris F, Gimenez R, Olalla M, Lopez MC. Mineral content in legumes and nuts: contribution to the Spanish dietary intake. *Sci Total Environ.* 2003, 308:1–14.

Campos-Vega R, Guevara-Gonzalez RG, Guevara-Olvera BL, Oomah BD, Loarca-Piña G. Bean (*Phaseolus vulgaris L.*) polysaccharides modulate gene expression in human colon cancer cells (HT-29.) *Food Res Intern.* 2010, 43:1057–1064.

Campos-Vega R, Reynoso-Camacho R, Pedraza-Aboytes G, Acosta-Gallegos JA, Guzman-Maldonado SH, Paredes-Lopez O, Oomah BD, Loarca-Piña G. Chemical composition and *in vitro* polysaccharide fermentation of different beans (*Phaseolus vulgaris* L.) *J Food Sci.* 2009, 74:59–65.

Carbonaro M, Grant G, Cappelloni M, Pusztai A. Perspectives into factors limiting *in vivo* digestion of legume proteins: antinutritional compounds or storage proteins? *J Agric Food Chem.* 2000, 48:742-749.

Cardador-Martinez A, Loarca-Pina G, Oomah BD. Antioxidant activity in common beans (*Phaseolus vulgaris* L.). *J Agric Food Chem.* 2002, 50:6975–80.

Castilla P, Echarri R, Davalos A, Cerrato F, Ortega H, Teruel JL, Lucas MF, Gomez-Coronado D, Ortuno J, Lasunción MA. Concentrated red grape juice exerts antioxidant, hypolipidemic, and antiinflammatory effects in both hemodialysis patients and healthy subjects. *Am J Clin Nutr.* 2006, 84:252–62.

Chai JW, Lim SL, Kanthimathi MS, Kuppusamy UR. Gene regulation in β-sitosterol-mediated stimulation of adipogenesis, glucose uptake, and lipid mobilization in rat primary adipocytes. *Genes Nutr.* 2011, 6(2):181-8.

Chanda S, Dudhatra S, Kaneria M. Antioxidative and antibacterial effects of seeds and fruit rind of nutraceutical plants belonging to the Fabaceae family. *Food Funct.* 2010, 1:308–315.

Chen C, Yu R, Owuor ED, Kong AN. Activation of antioxidant-response element (ARE), mitogen-activated protein kinases (MAPKs) and caspases by major green tea polyphenol components during cell survival and death. *Arch Pharm Res.* 2000, 23:605.

Chen CY. The noodle quality and physicochemical properties of various starches isolated by wet process. *MS thesis, National Taiwan University.* 1978.

Chen LH, Fang J, Sun Z, Li H, Wu Y, Demark-Wahnefried W, Lin X. Enterolactone inhibits insulin-like growth factor-1 receptor signaling in human prostatic carcinoma PC-3 cells. *J Nutr.* 2009, 139:653-659.

Chen Q, Liu S, Chen J, Zhang Q, Lin S, Chen Z, Jiang J. Luteolin induces mitochondria-dependent apoptosis in human lung adenocarcinoma cell *Nat Prod Commun.* 2012, 7(1):29-32.

Chen X, Krakauer T, Oppenheim JJ, Howard OM: An injectable multicomponent chinese herbal medicine, is a potent inhibitor of T-cell activation. *J Altern Complement Med.* 2004, 10:519-526.

Chien MH, Lee TS, Liang YC, Lee WS. β-Sitosterol inhibits cell cycle progression of rat aortic smooth muscle cells through increases of p21cip1 protein. *J Agric Food Chem.* 2010, 58(18):10064-10069.

Choi EJ, Kim GH. Daidzein causes cell cycle arrest at the G1 and G2/M phases in human breast cancer MCF-7 and MDA-MB-453 cells. *Phytomedicine.* 2008, 15:683-690.

Clemente A, Gee JM, Johnson IT, MacKenzie DA, Domoney C. Pea (*Pisum sativum*, L.) protease inhibitors from the Bowman-Birk class influence the growth of human colorectal adenocarcinoma HT29 cells *in vitro*. *J Agric Food Chem.* 2005, 53:8979-8986.

Constantinou AI, Lantvit D, Hawthorne M, et al Chemopreventive effects of soy protein and purified soy isoflavones on DMBA-induced mammary tumors in female Sprague–Dawley rats. *Nutr Cancer.* 2001, 41:75-81.

Costa de Almeida GE, Queiros Monici KS, Reis SMP, Costa de Oliviera A. Chemical composition, dietary fibre and resistant starch content of raw and cooked pea, common bean, chickpea and lentil legumes. *Food chem.* 2006, 94:327-330.

Coughlin CM, Salhany KE, Wysocka M, Aruga E, Kurzawa H, Chang AE, Hunter CA, Fox JC, Trinchieri G, Lee WM. Interleukin-12 and interleukin-18 synergistically induce murine tumor regression which involves inhibition of angiogenesis. J Clin Invest. 1998, 101:1441-*1452.*

Covas MI, Nyyssonen K, Poulsen HE, Kaikkonen J, Zunft HJ, Kiesewetter H, Gaddi A, de la Torre R, Mursu J, Bäumler H, Nascetti S, Salonen JT, Fitó M, Virtanen J, Marrugat J, EUROLIVE Study Group. The effect of polyphenols in olive oil on heart disease risk factors. *Ann Intern Med.* 2006;145:333–341.

Cuadrado C, Hajos G, Burbano C, Pedrosa MM, Ayet G, Muzquiz M, Puzstai A, Gelencser E. Effect of natural fermentation on the lectin of lentils measured by immunological methods. *Food Agric Immunol.* 2002, 14:41-44.

Cuevas-Martínez D, Moreno-Ramos C, Martínez-Manrique E, Moreno-Martínez E, Méndez-Albores A. Nutrition and texture evaluation of maize-white common bean nixtamalized tortillas. *Interciencia*. 2010, 35(11):828-832.

Dalgetty DD, Baik BK. Fortification of bread with hulls and cotyledon fibers isolated from peas, lentils and chickpeas. *Cereal Chem*. 2006, 83:269–274.

Dalgetty DD, Baik BK. Isolation and characterization of cotyledon fibers from peas, lentils, and chickpea. *Cereal Chem*. 2003, 80:310-315.

Davalos A, Fernandez-Hernando C, Cerrato F, Martinez-Botas J, Gomez-Coronado D, Gomez-Cordoves C, Lasuncion MA. Red grape juice polyphenols alter cholesterol homeostasis and increase LDL receptor activity in human cells in vitro. *J Nutr*. 2006, 136:1766–1773.

Davis MS, Miller CK, Mitchell DC. More favorable dietary patterns are associated with lower glycemic load in older adults. *J Am Diet Assoc*. 2004, 104:1828-1835.

de Almeida Costa GE, Queiroz-Monici KdS, Reis SMPM, Costa de Oliveira A. Chemical composition, dietary fibre and resistant starch contents of raw and cooked pea, common bean, chickpea and lentil legumes. *Food Chem*. 2006, 94:327–330.

de la Hera E, Ruiz-París E, Oliete B, Gómez M. Studies of the quality of cakes made with wheat-lentil composite flours LWT - *Food Sci Technology*. 2012, 49(1):48–54.

Dhingra S, Jood S. Organoleptic and nutritional evaluation of wheat breads supplemented with soybean and barley flour. *Food Chem*. 2001, 77:479-488.

Díaz-Batalla L, Widholm JM, Fahey CG, Castaño-Tostado E, Paredes-López O. Chemical components with health implications in wild and cultivated Mexican common bean seeds (*Phaseolus vulgaris* L.). *J Agric Food* Chem. 2006, 54:2045-2052.

Doblado R, Zielinski H, Piskula M, Kozlowska H, Muñoz R, Frías J, Vidal-Valverde C. Effect of processing on the antioxidant vitamins and antioxidant capacity of *Vigna sinensis* var. Carilla. *J Agric Food Chem*. 2005, 53:1215–1222.

Dreher ML, Patek JW. Effects of supplementation of short bread cookies with roasted whole navy bean flour and high protein flour. *J Food Sci*. 1984, 49(3):922–924.

Duane WC. Effects of legume consumption on serum cholesterol, biliary lipids, and sterol metabolism in humans. *J Lipid Res*. 1997, 38:1120-1128.

Duranti M. Grain legume proteins and nutraceutical properties. *Fitoterapia*. 2006, 77:67–82.

Dutta D, Chaudhuri UR, Chakraborty R. Structure, health benefits, antioxidant property and processing and storage of carotenoids. *Afr J Biotechnol*. 2005, 4(13):1510-1520.

Dziuba J, Minkiewicz P, Nalecz D. Biologically active peptides from plant and animal proteins. *Pol J Food Nutr Sci*. 1999, 8:3-16.

Dzudie T, Scher J, Hardy J. Common bean flour as an extender in beef sausages. *J Food Eng*. 2002, 52:143–147.

Edelenbos M, Christensen LP, Grevsen K. HPLC Determination of chlorophyll and carotenoid pigments in processed green pea cultivars (*Pisum sativum* L.). *J Agric Food Chem*. 2001, 49(10):4768–4774.

Eisenstein J, Roberts SB, Dallal G, Saltzman E. High-protein weight-loss diets: are they safe and do they work? A review of the experimental and epidemiologic data. *Nutr Rev* 2002, 60:189-200.

el-Deiry WS, Tokino T, Velculescu VE, Levy DB, Parsons R, Trent JM, Lin D, Mercer WE, Kinzler KW, Vogelstein B. WAF1, a potential mediator of p53 tumor suppression. Cell. 1993, 75:817-825.

Emenaker NJ, Calaf GM, Cox D, Basson MD, Qureshi N. Short-chain fatty acids inhibit invasive human colon cancer by modulating uPA, TIMP-1, TIMP-2, mutant p53, Bcl-2, Bax, p21 and PCNA protein expression in an *in vitro* cell culture model. *J Nutr.* 2001, 131:3041S–3046S.

Eriksson U, Danilczyk U, Penninger JM. Just the beginning: novel functions for angiotensinconverting enzymes. *Curr Biol.* 2002, 12:R745-R752.

Escudero-Álvarez E, González-Sánchez P. La fibra dietética. *Nutr Hosp.* 2006, 21(Supl.2):61-72.

Espinosa-Alonso LG, Lygin A, Wildholm JM, Valverde ME, Paredes-Lopez O. polyphenols in wild and weedy Mexican common beans (*Phaseolus vulgaris* L.). *J Agric Food Chem.* 2006, 54:4436-4444.

Fang MZ, Chen D, Sun Y, Jin Z, Christman JK, Yang CS. Reversal of hypermethylation and reactivation of p16INK4a, RARb, and MGMT genes by genistein and other isoflavones from soy. *Clin Cancer Res.* 2005, 11:7033-7041.

Feregrino-Pérez AA, Berumen LC, García-Alcocer G, Guevara-González RG, Ramos-Gómez M, Reynoso-Camacho R, Acosta-Gallegos JA, Loarca-Piña G. Composition and chemopreventive effect of polysaccharides from common beans (*Phaseolus vulgaris* L.) on Azoxymetane-induced colon cancer. *J Agric Food Chem.* 2008, 56:8737-8744.

Finkina KI, Shramova EI, Tagaev AA, Ovchinnikova TV. A novel defensin from the lentil (*Lens culinaris*) seeds. *Biochem Biophys Res Commun.* 2008, 371:860-865

Finley JW, Burrell JB, Reeves PG. Pinto bean consumption changes SCFA profiles in fecal fermentations, bacterial populations of the lower bowel, and lipid profiles in blood of humans. *J Nutr.* 2007, 137: 2391–2398.

Foster-Powell K, Miller JB. International tables of glycemic index. *Am J Clin Nutr.* 1995, 62(suppl):871S-890S.

Fotsis T, Pepper M, Adlercreutz H, Hase T, Montesano R, Schweigerer L. Genistein, a dietary ingested isoflavonoid, inhibits cell proliferation and *in vitro* angiogenesis. *J Nutr.* 1995, 125:790S–797S.

Fresco P, Borges F, Marques MPM, Diniz C. The anticancer properties of dietary polyphenols and its relation with apoptosis. *Curr Pharm Des.* 2010, 16: 114-134.

Fruhbeck G, Monreal I, Santidrian S. Hormonal implications of the hypocholesterolemic effect of intake of field beans (*Vicia faba* L.) by young men with hypercholesterolemia. *Am J Clin Nutr.* 1997, 66:1452–1460.

Fu, YH, Zhang, FC. Changes in isoflavone glucoside and aglycone contents of chickpea yogurth during fermentation by lactobacillus bulgaricus and streptococcus thermophilus. *J Food Process Preservation.* 2012, doi: 10.1111/j.1745-4549.2012.00713.x

Fujita H, Yokoyama K, Yoshikawa M. Classification and antihypertensive activity of angiotensin I-converting enzyme inhibitory peptides derived from food proteins. *J Food Sci.* 2000, 65:564–569.

Gálvez-Ranilla L, Genovese MI, Lajolo FM. Polyphenols and antioxidant capacity of seed coat and cotyledon from Brazilian and Peruvian bean cultivars (*Phaseolus vulgaris* L.). *J Agric Food Chem.* 2007, 55:90-98.

García-Gasca T, Salazar-Olivo LA, Mendiola-Olaya E, Blanco-Labra A. The effects of a protease inhibitor fraction from tepary bean (*Phaseolus acutifolius*) on *in vitro* cell proliferation and cell adhesion of transformed cells. *Toxicol In Vitro.* 2002, 16:229–233.

Garrido C, Gurbuxani S, Ravagnan L, Kroemer G. Heat shock proteins: endogenous modulators of apoptotic cell death. *Biochem Biophys Res Commun.* 2001, 286:433-442.

Geraedts MC, Troost FJ, Saris WH. Addition of sucralose enhances the release of satiety hormones in combination with pea protein. Mol Nutr Food Res. 2012, 56(3):417-424.

Geraedts MCP, Troost FJ, Munsters MJM, Stegen JHCH, de Ridder RJ, Conchillo JM, Kruimel JW, Masclee AAM, Saris WHM. Intraduodenal administration of intact pea protein effectively reduces food intake in both lean and obese male subjects. *PLoS ONE.* 2011, 6(9):e24878.

Gerald RJ, Murray BA, Walsh DJ. Hypotensive peptides from milk proteins. *J Nutr.* 2004, 134: 980S–988S.

Gercel-Taylor C, Feitelson AK, Taylor DD. Inhibitory effect of genistein and daidzein on ovarian cancer cell growth. *Anticancer Res.* 2004, 24:795-800.

Gómez M, Oliete B, Rosell CM, Pando V, Fernández E. Studies on cake quality made of wheat-chickpea flour blends. *LWT-Food Sci Technology.* 2008, 41(9): 1701-1709.

Goni I, Valentin-Gamazo C. Chickpea flour ingredient slows glycemic response to pasta in healthy volunteers. *Food Chem.* 2002, 81:511-515.

González de Mejía E, Guzmán-Maldonado SH, Acosta-Gallegos JA, Reynoso-Camacho R, Ramírez-Rodríguez E, Pons-Hernández JL, González-Chavira MM, Castellanos JZ, Kelly JD. Effect of cultivar and growing location on the trypsin inhibitors, tannins, and lectins of common beans (*Phaseolus vulgaris* L.) grown in the semiarid highlands of Mexico. *J. Agric Food Chem.* 2003, 51:5962-5966.

González de Mejía E, Prisecaru VI. Lectins as bioactive plant proteins: A potential in cancer treatment. *Crit Rev Food Sci Nutr.* 2005, 45:425–445.

González de Mejía E, Valdez-Vega MC, Reynoso-Camacho R, Loarca-Piña G. Tannins, trypsin inhibitors and lectin cytotoxicity in tepary (*Phaseolus acutifolius*) and common (*Phaseolus vulgaris*) beans. *Plant Foods Human Nutr.* 2005, 60:137-145.

Granado-Serrano AB, Martín MA, Haegeman G, Goya L, Bravo L, Ramos S. Epicatechin induces NF-kappaB, activator protein-1 (AP-1) and nuclear transcription factor erythroid 2p45-related factor-2 (Nrf2) via phosphatidylinositol-3-kinase/protein kinase B (PI3K/AKT) and extracellular regulated kinase (ERK) signalling in HepG2 cells. *Br J Nutr.* 2010, 103(2):168-179.

Granito M, Champ M, David A, Bonnet C, Guerra M. Identification of gas-producing components in different varieties of *Phaseolus vulgaris* by *in vitro* fermentation. *J Sci Food Agric.* 2001, 81:543-550.

Granito M, Trujillo L, Guerra M. Use of *Phaseolus vulgaris* and *Vigna sinensis* in a fermented dairy drink. *Arch Latinoam Nutr.* 2004, 54(2):229-234.

Granito M, Valero Y, Zambrano R. Baked product development based fermented legumes and cereals for school children snack. *Arch Latinoam Nutr.* 2010, 60(1):85-92.

Gudbrandsen OA, Wergedahl H, Mork S, Liaset B, Espe M, Berge RK. Dietary soya protein concentrate enriched with isoflavones reduced fatty liver, increased hepatic fatty acid oxidation and decreased the hepatic mRNA level of VLDL receptor in obese Zucker rats. *Br J Nutr.* 2006, 96:249–257.

Guo JM, Xiao BX, Dai DJ, Liu Q, Ma HH. Effects of daidzein on estrogen-receptor-positive and negative pancreatic cancer cells *in vitro*. *World J Gastroenterol.* 2004a, 10(6):860-863.

Guo JM, Xiao BX, Liu DH, Grant M, Zhang S, Lai YF, Guo YB, Liu Q. Biphasic effect of daidzein on cell growth of human colon cancer cells. *Food Chem Toxicol.* 2004b, 42:1641-1646.

Guzik TJ, West NE, Black E, McDonald D, Ratnatunga C, Pillai R, Channon KM. Vascular superoxide production by NAD(P)H oxidase: association with endothelial dysfunction and clinical risk factors. *Circ Res.* 2000, 86:E85–E90.

Hague A, Manning A, Hanlon K, Huschtscha LI, Hart D, Paraskeva C. Sodium butyrate induces apoptosis in human colonic tumor cell lines in a p53 independent pathway: implications for the possible role of dietary fiber in the prevention of large bowel cancer. *Int J Cancer.* 1993, 55:498-505.

Han J, Inaguma T, Isoda H. Cyanidin 3-glucoside anthocyanin from black beans has potential to protect insulin resistance on 3T3-L1 adipocytes by inhibiting TNF-α release. *Br J Nutr.* 2012, *In press.*

Han J, Janz J, Gerlat M. Development of gluten-free cracker snacks using pulse flours and fractions. *Food Res Int.* 2010, 43:627–633.

Han KH, Iijuka M, Shimada K, Sekikawa M, Kuramochi K, Ohba K, Ruvini L, Chiji H, Fukushima M. Adzuki resistant starch lowered serum cholesterol and hepatic 3-hydroxy-3-methylglutaryl-CoA mRNA levels and increased hepatic LDL-receptor and cholesterol 7α-hydroxylase mRNA levels in rats fed a cholesterol diet. *Br J Nutr.* 2006, 94(6):902–908.

Han KH, Sekikawa M, Shimada KI, Sasaki K, Ohba K, Fukushima M. Resistant starch fraction prepared from kintoki bean affects gene expression of genes associated with cholesterol metabolism in rats. *Exp Biol Med.* 2004, 229:787-792.

Hangen L, Bennink MR. Consumption of black beans and navy beans (*Phaseolus vulgaris*) reduced azoxymethane-induced colon cancer in rats. *Nutr Cancer.* 2002, 44(1):60-65.

Hargreaves DF, Potten CS, Harding C, Shaw LE, Morton MS, Roberts SA, Howell A, Bundred NJ. Two-week dietary soy supplementation has an estrogenic effect on normal premenopausal breast. *J Clin Endocrinol Metab.* 1999, 84:4017–4024.

Harland J. Prevention is better than cure (soy isoflavones). *Liquid Food Drink Technol,* 2002, 1.

Harper CE, Cook LM, Patel BB, Wang J, Eltoum IA, Arabshahi A, Shirai T, Lamartiniere CA. Genistein and resveratrol, alone and in combination, suppress prostate cancer in SV-40 tag rats. *Prostate.* 2009, 69(15):1668–1682.

Hawkins A, Johnson SK. *In vitro* carbohydrate digestibility of whole chickpea and chickpea bread products. *Int J Food Sci Nutr.* 2005, 56:147-155.

Hodek P, Trefil P, Stiborova M: Flavonoids-potent and versatile biologically active compounds interacting with cytochromes P450. *Chem Biol Interact.* 2002, 139.1-21.

Hoojjat P, Zabik ME. Sugar-Snap cookies prepared with wheat-navy bean-sesame seed flour blends. *Cereal Chem.* 1984, 61(1):41-44.

Hou DX, Kumamoto T. Flavonoids as protein kinase inhibitors for cancer chemoprevention: Direct binding and molecular modeling. *Antioxid Redox Signal.* 2010, 13(5):691-719.

Hsu CC, Lin TW, Chang WW, Wu CY, Lo WH, Wang PH, Tsai YC. Soyasaponin-I-modified invasive behavior of cancer by changing cell surface sialic acids. *Gynecol Oncol.* 2005, 96(2):415-422.

Hu R, Kong ANT. Activation of MAP kinases, apoptosis and nutrigenomics of gene expression elicited by dietary cancer-prevention compounds. *Nutrition.* 2004, 20:83–88.

Li H, Prairie N, Udenigwe CC, Adebiyi AP, Tappia PS, Aukema HM, Jones PJH, Aluko RE. Blood pressure lowering effect of a pea protein hydrolysate in hypertensive rats and humans. *J Agric Food Chem.* 2011, 59: 9854–9860.

Huh JE, Nam DW, Baek YH, Kang JW, Park DS, Choi DY, Lee JD. Formononetin accelerates wound repair by the regulation of early growth response factor-1 transcription factor through the phosphorylation of the ERK and p38 MAPK pathways. *Int Immunopharmacol.* 2011, 1:46-54.

Ibrikci H, Knewtson SJB, Grusak MA. Chickpea leaves as a vegetable green for humans: Evaluation of mineral composition. *J Sci Food Agric.* 2003, 83:945-950.

Inaguma T, Han J, Isoda H. Improvement of insulin resistance by cyanidin 3-glucoside, anthocyanin from black beans through the up-regulation of GLUT4 gene expression. *BMC Proc.* 2011, 5(Suppl 8):P21.

Iqbal A, Khalil A, Ateeq N, Khan MS. Nutritional quality of important food legumes. *Food Chem.* 2006, 97:331-335.

Iqbal MJ, Yaegashi S, Ahsan R, Lightfoot DA, Banz WJ. Differentially abundant mRNAs in rat liver in response to diets containing soy protein isolate. *Physiol Genomics.* 2002, 11:219–226.

Jenab M, Thompson LU. Role of phytic acid in cancer and other diseases. *In*: *Food Phytates.* Reddy, N. R., Sathe, S. K., Eds., CRC Press: Boca Raton, FL, 2002. Pp. 225-248.

Jenkins DJ, Kendall CW, Augustin LS, Franceschi S, Hamidi M, Marchie A, Jenkins AL, Axelsen M. Glycemic index: overview of implications in health and disease. *Am J Clin Nutr.* 2002, 76:266S-273S.

Jesch ED, Seo JM, Carr TP, Lee JY. Sitosterol reduces messenger RNA and protein expression levels of Niemann-Pick C1-like 1 in FHs 74 Int cells. *Nutr Res.* 2009, 29(12):859-866.

Jin S, Zhang QY, Kang XM, Wang JX, Zhao WH. Daidzein induces MCF-7 breast cancer cell apoptosis via the mitochondrial pathway. *Ann Oncol.* 2010, 2:263-268.

Jin Z, MacDonald RS. Soy isoflavones increase latency of spontaneous mammary tumors in mice. *J Nutr.* 2002, 132:3186-3190.

Johnson SK, Thomas SJ, Hall RS. Potability and glucose, insulin and satiety responses of chickpea flour and extruded chickpea flour bread eaten as part of a breakfast. *Eur J Clin Nutr.* 2005, 59:169-176.

Jood S, Bishnoi S, Sharma A. Chemical analysis and physicochemical properties of chickpea and lentil cultivars. *Nahrung/Food.* 1998, 42:71–74.

Ju YH, Fultz J, Allred KF, Doerge DR, Helferich WG. Effects of dietary daidzein and its metabolite, equol, at physiological concentrations on the growth of estrogen-dependent human breast cancer (MCF-7) tumors implanted in ovariectomized athymic mice. *Carcinogenesis.* 2006, 27:856-863.

Kabagambe EK, Baylin A, Ruiz-Narvarez E, Siles X, Campos H. Decreased consumption of dried mature beans is positively associated with urbanization and nonfatal acute myocardial infarction. *J Nutr.* 2005, 135(7):1770-1775.

Kaldas RS, Hughes CL Jr. Reproductive and general metabolic effects of phytoestrogens in mammals. *Reprod Toxicol.* 1989, 3:81–89.

Kan A, Özçelik B, Kartal M. *In vitro* antiviral activities under cytotoxic doses against *herpes simples* type-1 and *parainfluensa*-3 viruses of *Cicer arietinum* L. (Chickpea) *Afr J Ph Pharm.* 2009, 3(12):627-631.

Kanamoto Y, Yamashita Y, Nanba F, Yoshida T, Tsuda T, Fukuda I, Nakamura-Tsuruta S, Ashida H. A black soybean seed coat extract prevents obesity and glucose intolerance by up-regulating uncoupling proteins and down-regulating inflammatory cytokines in high-fat diet-fed mice. *J Agric Food Chem.* 2011, 59:8985–8993.

Kapral M, Wawszczyk J, Jurzak M, Hollek A, Weglarz L. The effect of inositol hepaphosphate on the expression of selected metalloproteinases and their tissue inhibitors in IL-β-stimulated colon cancer cells. *Int J Colorectal Dis.* 2012, DOI 10.1007/s00384-012-1445-3.

Kasimanickam RK, Kasimanickam VR. Effect of tocopherol supplementation on serum 8-epi-prostaglandin F2 alpha and adiponectin concentrations, and mRNA expression of PPARγ and related genes in ovine placenta and uterus. *Theriogenology.* 2011, 76(3):482-491.

Kempuraj D, Tagen M, Iliopoulou BP, Clemons A, Vasiadi M, Boucher W, House M, Wolfberg A, Theoharides TC: Luteolin inhibits myelin basic protein-induced human mast cell activation and mast cell-dependent stimulation of Jurkat T cells. *Br J Pharmacol.* 2008, 155:1076-1084.

Kennedy AR, Billings PC, Wan XS, Newberne PM. Effects of Bowman-Birk inhibitor on rat colon carcinogenesis. *Nutr Cancer.* 2002, 43(2):174–186.

Khan N, Afaq F, Mukhtar H. Cancer chemoprevention through dietary antioxidants: progress and promise. *Antioxid Redox Signal.* 2008, 10:475-510.

Kim YS, Wiesenborn DP, Lorenzen JH, Berglund P. Suitability of edible bean and potato starches for starch noodles. *Cereal Chem.* 1996, 73(3):302-308.

Knott RM, Grant G, Bardocz S, Pusztai A, de Carvalh AFFU, Hexeth IH Alterations in the level of insulin receptor and GLUT-4 mRNA in skeletal muscle from rats fed a kidney bean (*Phaseolus vulgaris*) diet. *Int J Biochem.* 1992, 24(6):897-902.

Kole L, Giri B, Manna SK, Pal B, Ghosh S. Biochanin-A, an isoflavon, showed anti-proliferative and anti-inflammatory activities through the inhibition of iNOS expression, p38-MAPK and ATF-2 phosphorylation and blocking NFκB nuclear translocation. *Eur J Pharmacol.* 2011, 653(1-3):8-15.

Krezowski PA, Nuttall FQ, Gannon MC, Billington CJ, Parker S. Insulin and glucose responses to various starch-containing foods in type II diabetic subjects. *Diabetes Care.* 1987, 10:205-212.

Krupa-Kozak U, Juskiewicz J, Wronkowska M, Soral-Smietana M, Zdunczyk Z. Native and microwaved bean and pea starch preparations: physiological effects on the intestinal ecosystem, caecal tissue and serum lipids in rats. *Br J Nutr.* 2010, 103:1118–1126.

Kumar U, Chen J, Sapoznikhov V, Canteros G, White BH, Sidhu A. Overexpression of inducible nitric oxide synthase in the kidney of the spontaneously hypertensive rat. *Clin Exp Hypertens.* 2005, 27:17–31.

Kuo SM. Antiproliferative potency of structurally distinct dietary flavonoids on human colon cancer cells. *Cancer Lett.* 1996, 110:41.

Lam SK, Ng TB. Apoptosis of human breast cancer cells induced by hemagglutinin from *Phaseolus vulgaris* cv. *Legumi secchi. Food Chem.* 2011, 126:595–602.

Lazarevic B, Boezelijn G, Diep LM. Efficacy and safety of short-term genistein intervention in patients with localized prostate cancer prior to radical prostatectomy: a randomized, placebo-controlled, double-blind Phase 2 clinical trial. *Nutr Cancer.* 2011, 6:889–898.

Li S, Yang S. IP-6 Induces apoptosis and enhances expression of Cspase 3 in HT-29 human colon carcinoma cell line. *Acta Academiae Medicine Qingdao Universitatis.* 2008-03.

Liener IE. Implications of antinutritional components in soybean foods. *Crit Rev Food Sci Nutr.* 1994, 34:31–67.

Lii CY, Chang SM. Characterization of red bean (*Phaseolus radiatus* var. Aurea) starch and its noodle quality. *J Food Sci.* 1981, 46(1):78-81.

Longnecker N, Kelly R, Huang S. (2002). The lentil lifestyle: Health benefits of lentils and their uses in diets. In Proceedings of lentil focus 2002, *National conference,* Horsham, (Victoria) (pp. 58–59).

Losso JN. The biochemical and functional food properties of the Bowman-Birk inhibitor. *Crit Rev Food Sci Nutr.* 2008, 4:94-118.

Luhovyy BL, Akhavan T, Anderson GH: Whey proteins in the regulation of food intake and satiety. *J Am Coll Nutr.* 2007, 26:704S-712S.

Maaroufi C, Melcion JP, Monredon F, Giboulot B, Guibert D, Le Guen MP. Fractionation of pea flour with pilot scale sieving. I. Physical and chemical characteristics of pea seed fractions. *Animal Feed Sci Technology.* 2000, 85:61-78.

Maccaferri S, Klinder A, Cacciatore S, Chitarrari R, Honda H, Luchinat C, Bertini I, Carnevali P, Gibson GR, Brigidi P, Costabile A. *In vitro* fermentation of potential prebiotic flours from natural sources: Impact on the human colonic microbiota and metabolome. *Mol Nutr Food Res.* 2012, doi: 10.1002/mnfr.201200046.

Manna SK Double-edged sword effect of biochanin to inhibit nuclear factor kappaB: suppression of serine/threonine and tyrosine kinases. *Biochem Pharmacol.* 2012, 83(10):1383-1392.

Marco C, Rosell CM. Functional and rheological properties of protein enriched gluten free composite flours. *J Food Eng,* 2008, 88(1):94–103.

Mariadason JM, Georgia AC, Augenlicht LH. Genetic reprogramming in pathways of colonic cell maturation induced by short chain fatty acids: comparison with trichostatin A, sulindac, and curcumin and implications for chemeprevention of colon cancer. *Cancer Res.* 2000, 60:4561–4572.

Marino E, Cardier JE. Differential effect of IL-18 on endothelial cell apoptosis mediated by TNF-alpha and Fas (CD95). Cytokine. 2003, 22*:*142-*148.*

Marles MS, Warkentin TD, Bett KE. Genotypic abundance of carotenoids and polyphenolics in the hull of field pea (*Pisum sativum* L.*) J Sci Food Agric.* 2012, doi: 10.1002/jsfa.5782

Marzo F, Alonso R, Urdaneta E, Arricibita FJ, Ibáñez F. Nutritional quality of extruded kidney bean (*Phaseolus vulgaris* L. var. Pinto) and its effects on growth and skeletal muscle nitrogen fractions in rats. *J Anim Sci.* 2002, 80:875–879.

Mathers JC. Pulses and carcinogenesis: potential for the prevention of colon, breast and other cancers. *Br J Nutr.* 2002, 88(3):S273–S279.

McCullough ML, Giovannucci EL. Diet and cancer prevention. *Oncogene.* 2004, 23:6349-6364.

McWatters KH. Replacement of milk protein with protein from cowpea and field pea flours in baking powder biscuits. *Cereal Chem.* 1980, 57(3):223-226.

Meisel H. Biochemical properties of regulatory peptides derived from milk proteins. *Biopolymers.* 1997, 43:119–128.

Mejia EGL, Prisecaru VI. Lectins as bioactive plant proteins: a potential in cancer treatment. *Critic Rev Food Sci Nutr.* 2005, 45:425-445.

Messina MJ. Legumes and soybeans: overview of their nutritional profiles and health effects. *Am J Clin Nutr.* 1999, 70:439S-450S.

Meuser F. Technological aspects of dietary fibre. In: McCleary, B.V., Prosky, L. (Eds.), *Advanced dietary fibre technology.* Blackwell Science, Oxford, 2001, pp. 248–269.

Mills PK, Beeson WL, Phillips RL, Fraser GE. Cohort study of diet, lifestyle, and prostate-cancer in adventist men. *Cancer.* 1989, 64(3):598-604.

Miñarro B, Albanell E, Aguilara N, Guamis B, Capellas M. Effect of legume flours on baking characteristics of gluten-free bread. *J Cereal Sci.* 2012, 56 (2): 476-481.

Mintel. *Frozen and canned fruit and vegetables – UK. Mintel Reports – UK series.* Mintel Group. 2005.

Modi VK, Mahendrakar NS, Rao DN, Sachindra NM. Quality of buffalo meat burger containing legume flours as binders. *Meat Sci.* 2004, 66(1):143–149.

Mohammeda I, Ahmeda AR, Senge B. Dough rheology and bread quality of wheat–chickpea flour blends. *Ind Crops Prod.* 2012, 36(1):196–202.

Moon DO, Kim MO, Choi YH, Kim GY. Beta-sitosterol induces G2/M arrest, endoreduplication, and apoptosis through the Bcl-2 and PI3K/Akt signaling pathways. *Cancer Lett.* 2008, 264(2):181-191.

Mora-Avilés A, Lemus-Flores B, Miranda-López R, Hernández-López D, Pons-Hernández JL, Acosta-Gallegos JA, Guzmán-Maldonado SH. Effects of common bean enrichment on nutritional quality of tortillas produced from nixtamalized regular and quality protein maize flours. *J Sci Food Agr.* 2007, 87(5): 880–886.

Morrow B. The rebirth of legumes: legume production, consumption and export are increasing as more people become aware of legumes nutritional benefits. *Food Technol.* 1991, 9:96–121.

Mueller SO. Overview of *in vitro* tools to assess the estrogenic and antiestrogenic activity of phytoestrogens. *J Chromatogr B Analyt Technol Biomed Life Sci.* 2002, 777: 155–165.

Mukai Y, Sato S. Polyphenol-containing azuki bean (*Vigna angularis*) seed coats attenuate vascular oxidative stress and inflammation in spontaneously hypertensive rats. *J Nutr Biochem. 2011*, 22:16–21.

Murakami T, Kohno K, Matsuda H, Yoshikawa M. Medicinal Foodstuffs. XXV.1 Hepatoprotective principle and structures of ionone glucoside, phenethyl glycoside, and flavonol oligoglycosides from young seedpods of garden peas, *Pisum sativum* L. *Chem Pharm Bull.* 2001b, 49:73—77.

Murakami T, Kohno K, Matsuda H, Yoshikawa M. Medicinal Foodstuffs. XXII. Structures of oleanane-type triterpene oligoglycosides, pisumsaponins I and II, and kaurane-type diterpene oligoglycosides, pisumosides A and B, from green peas, the immature seeds of *Pisum sativum* L. *Chem Pharm Bull.* 2001b, 49(1):73-77.

Muzquiz M, Burbano C, Ayet G, Pedrosa MM, Cuadrado C. The investigation of antinutritional factors in *Phaseolus vulgaris*. Environmental and varietal differences. *Biotechnol Agron Soc Environ.* 1999, 3(4):210–216.

Newgent J. Nutrition guide: is folate on your plate? Heart Information Network. 2001. http://www.heartinfo.org/nutrition/folate4398.htm

Niba LL, Niba SN. Role of non-digestible carbohydrates in colon cancer protection. *Nutr Food Sci.* 2003, 33(1):28-33.

Nilsson J, Stegmark R, Åkessen B. Total antioxidant capacity in different pea (*Pisum sativum*) varieties after blanching and freezing. *Food Chem.* 2004, 86:501–507.

Oboh HA, Omofoma CO. The effects of heat treated lima beans (*Phaseolus lunatus*) on plasma lipids in hypercholesterolemic rats. *Pakistan J Nutr.* 2008, 7(5):636-639.

Oomah BD, Cardador-Martinez A, Loarca-Pina G. Phenolics and antioxidative activities in common beans (*Phaseolus vulgaris* L.). *J Sci Food Agric.* 2005, 85:935–942.

Oomah BD, Corbé A, Balasubramanian PM. Antioxidant and anti-inflammatory activities of bean (*Phaseolus vulgaris* L.) hulls. *J Agric Food Chem.* 2010, 58(14):8225-8230.

Pages F, Berger A, Henglein B, Piqueras B, Danel C, Zinzindohoue F, Thiounn N, Cugnenc PH, Fridman WH. Modulation of interleukin-18 expression in human colon carcinoma: consequences for tumor immune surveillance. *Int J Cancer.* 1999, 84*:326-330.*

Pelembe L, Erasmus C, Taylor R. Development of a protein rich composite sorghum–cowpea instant porridge by extrusion cooking process. *Lebensm -Wiss Technol.* 2002, 35:120–127.

Perabo FGE, Von Löw EC, Ellinger J, von R¨ucker A, Müller SC, Bastian PJ. Soy isoflavone genistein in prevention and treatment of prostate cancer. *Prostate Cancer and Prostatic Dis.* 2008, 1:6–12.

Petitot M, Boyer L, Minier C, Micard V. Fortification of pasta with split pea and faba bean flours: pasta processing and quality evaluation. *Food Res Int.* 2010, 43:634–641.

Pietrasik Z, Janz JAM. Utilization of pea flour, starch-rich and fiber-rich fractions in low fat bologna. *Food Res Int.* 2010, 43:602–608.

Pittaway JK, Ahuja KDK, Robertson LK, Ball MJ. Effect of controlled diet supplemented with chickpeas on serum lipids, glucose tolerance, satiety and bowel function. *J Am Coll Nutr.* 2007, 26:334-340.

Po LS, Chen ZY, Tsang DS, Leung LK. Baicalein and genistein display differential actions on estrogen receptor (ER) transactivation and apoptosis in MCF-7 cells. *Cancer Lett.* 2002, 187: 33–40.

Pryme IF, Bardocz S, Pusztai A, Ewen SW. The growth of an established murine non-Hodgkin lymphoma tumour is limited by switching to a phytohaemagglutinin-containing diet. *Cancer Lett.* 1999, 146(1):87-91.

Qiao H, Zhang X, Zhu C, Dong L, Wang L, Zhang X, Xing Y, Wang C, Ji Y, Cao X. Luteolin downregulates TLR4, TLR5, NF-κB and p-p38MAPK expression, upregulates the p-ERK expression, and protects rat brains against focal ischemia. *Brain Res.* 2012, 1448:71-81.

Rafter J. Lactic acid bacteria and cancer: mechanistic perspective. *Br J Nutr.* 2002, 88(Suppl. 1):S89–S94.

Raines EW, Ross R. Biology of atherosclerotic plaque formation: possible role of growth factors in lesion development and the potential impact of soy. *J Nutr.* 1995, 125:624S–630S.

Rao AV, Rao LG. Carotenoids and human health. *Pharmacol Res.* 2007, 55:207–216.

Ravindran G, Gamlath S. Functional extruded snack products based on chickpea (*Cicer arietinum* L.) and fenugreek (*Trigonella foenum-graecum*) flours, in NZNS & NSA 2007: *Joint New Zealand Nutrition Society and Nutrition Society of Australia Annual Scientific Meeting,* Nutrition Society of Australia, Kent Town, S. Aust.

Richter M, Ebermann R, Marian B. Quercetin-induced apoptosis in colorectal tumor cells: possible role of EGF receptor signaling. *Nutr Cancer.* 1999, 34(1):88-99.

Rigamonti E, Parolini C, Marchesi M, Diani E, Brambilla S, Sirtori CR Chiesa G. Hypolipidemic effect of dietary pea proteins: Impact on genes regulating hepatic lipid metabolism. *Mol Nutr Food Res.* 2010, 54:S24–S30.

Rijken PJ, Timmer WG, van de Kooij AJ, van Benschop IM, Wiseman SA, Meijers M, Tijburg LBM. Effect of vegetable and carotenoid consumption on aberrant crypt multiplicity, a surrogate end-point marker for colorectal cancer in azoxymethane-induced rats. *Carcinogensis.* 1999, 20(12):2267-2272.

Rimm EB, Ascherio A, Giovannucci E, Spiegelman D, Stampfer MJ, Willett WC. Vegetable, fruit and cereal fiber intake and risk of coronary heart disease among men. *JAMA.* 1996, 275:447-451.

Rodríguez-Castillo L, Fernández XE. Los frijoles (*Phaseolus vulgaris*): su aporte a la dieta del costarricense. *Acta Med Costar.* 2003, 45(3):120-125.

Rozza L, Hiruma-Lima CA, Tanimoto A, Pellizzon CH. Morphologic and pharmacological investigations in the epicatechin gastroprotective effect. *Evid Based Complement Med.* 2012, doi:10.1155/2012/708156.

Saied IT, Shamsuddin AM. Up-regulation of the tumor suppressor gene p53 and WAF1 gene expression by IP6 in HT-29 human colon carcinoma cell line. *Anticancer Res.* 1998, 18:1479–1484.

Salvemini D. Superoxide: a key player in hypertension. *FASEB J.* 2004, 18:94–101.

Sanchez M, Galisteo M, Vera R,Villar IC, Zarzuelo A, Tamargo J, Pérez-Vizcaíno F, Duarte J. Quercetin downregulates NADPH oxidase, increases eNOS activity and prevents endothelial dysfunction in spontaneously hypertensive rats. *J Hypertens.* 2006, 24:75–84.

Santti R, Makela S, Strauss L, Korkman J, Kostian ML. Phytoestrogens: potential endocrine disruptors in males. *Toxicol Ind Health.* 1998, 14:223–237.

Sanz Y, Collado MC, Haros M, Dalmau J. Funciones metabólico nutritivas de la microbiota intestinal y su modulación a través de la dieta: probióticos y prebióticos. *Acta Pediatr Esp.* 2004, 62:520-526.

Sarnak MJ, Levey AS, Schoolwerth AC, Coresh J, Culleton B, Hamm LL, McCullough PA, Kasiske BL, Kelepouris E, Klag MJ, Parfrey P, Pfeffer M, Raij L, Spinosa DJ, Wilson PW. Kidney disease as a risk factor for development of cardiovascular disease: a statement from the American Heart Association Councils on Kidney in cardiovascular disease, high blood pressure research, clinical cardiology, and epidemiology and prevention. *Circulation.* 2003, 108: 2154–2169.

Sarr M, Chataigneau M, Martins S, Schott C, El Bedoui J, Oak MH, Muller B, Chataiqneau T, Schini-Kerth VB. Red wine polyphenols prevent angiotensin II-induced hypertension and endothelial dysfunction in rats: role of NADPH oxidase. *Cardiovasc Res.* 2006, 71:794–802.

Sathyamoorthy N, Wang TT. Differential effects of dietary phyto-oestrogens daidzein and equol on human breast cancer MCF-7 cells. *Eur J Cancer.* 1997, 33:2384–2389.

Selhub J, Jacques PF, Wilson PWF, Rush D, Rosenberg IH. Vitamin status and intake as primary determinants of homocysteinemia in an elderly population. *JAMA.* 1993, 270:2693-2698.

Sengupta S, Muir JG, Gibson PR. Does butyrate protect from colorectal cancer? *Review. J Gastroen Hepatol.* 2006, 21:209–218.

Serrano J, Goñi I. Papel del frijol negro *Phaseolus vulgaris* en el estado nutricional de la población guatemalteca. *Arch Latinoam Nutr.* 2004, 54(1):36-44.

Setchell KD, Brown NM, Lydeking-Olsen E. The clinical importance of the metabolite equol- a clue to the effectiveness of soy and its isoflavones. *J Nutr.* 2002, 132:3577–3584.

Shahzadi N, Butt MS, Rehman SU, Sharif K. Rheological and baking characters of composite flours. *Int J Agri Biol.* 2005, 7(1):100-104.

Shamsuddin AM, Ullah A. Inositol hexaphosphate inhibits large intestinal cancer in F344 rats 5 months after induction by azoxymethane. *Carcinogenesis.* 1989, 10:625–626.

Smulikowska S, Pastuszewska B, Swiech E, Ochtabinska A, Mieczkowska A, NguyenVC. Buraczewska L. Tannin content affects negatively nutritive value of pea for monogastrics. *J Anim Feed Sci.* 2001, 10:511-523.

Sotomayor C, Frias J, Vidal-Valverde C, Fornal J, Sadowska J, Urbano, G. Lentil starch content and its microscopical structure as influenced by natural fermentation. *Starch.* 1999, 51:152–156.

Spielmann J, Stangl GI, Eder K. Dietary pea protein stimulates bile acid excretion and lowers hepatic cholesterol concentration in rats. *J Anim Physiol Anim Nutr.* 2008, 683–693.

Stadelmann C. Recent advances in the neuropathology of multiple sclerosis. *J Neurochem* 2007, 163:657-661.

Sternberg Z, Chadha K, Lieberman A, Drake A, Hojnacki D, Weinstock-Guttman B, Munschauer F. Immunomodulatory responses of peripheral blood mononuclear cells from multiple sclerosis patients upon *in vitro* incubation with the flavonoid luteolin: additive effects of IFN-beta. *J Neuroinflammation.* 2009, (13)6:28 doi:10.1186/1742-2094-6-28.

Suzuki K, Koike H, Matsui H, Ono Y, Hasumi M, Nakazato H, Okugi H, Sekine Y, Oki K, Ito K, Yamamoto T, Fukabori Y, Kurokawa K, Yamanaka H. Genistein, a soy isoflavone, induces glutathione peroxidase in the human prostate cancer cell lines LNCaP and PC-3. *Int J Cancer.* 2002, 99(6):846-852.

Taniyama Y, Griendling KK. Reactive oxygen species in the vasculature: molecular and cellular mechanisms. *Hypertension.* 2003, 42:1075–1081.

Taylor WG, Richards KW. *Plant compositions enriched in dehydrosoyasaponin I (D-I) and methods of producing such compositions.* US Patent App. 12/522,436, 2007.

Theoharides TC, Kempuraj D, Kourelis T, Manola A: Human mast cells stimulate activated T cells: implications for multiple sclerosis. *Ann N Y Acad Sci.* 2008, 1144:74-82.

Thompson MD, Mensack MM, Jiang W, Zhu Z, Lewis MR, McGinley JN, Brick MA, Thompson HJ. Cell signaling pathways associated with a reduction in mammary cancer burden by dietary common bean (*Phaseolus vulgaris* L.). *Carcinogenesis.* 2012, 33(1):226–232.

Tiwari BK, Brennan CS, Jaganmohan R, Surabi A, Alagusundaram K. Utilisation of pigeon pea (*Cajanus cajan* L) byproducts in biscuit manufacture. *LWT- Food Sci Technol.* 2011, 44(6):1533–1537.

Torruco-Uco J, Chel-Guerrero L, Martínez-Ayala A, Dávila-Ortíz G, Betancur-Ancona D. Angiotensin-I converting enzyme inhibitory and antioxidant activities of protein hydrolysates from *Phaseolus lunatus* and *Phaseolus vulgaris* seeds. *Food Sci Technol.* 2009, 42:1597–1604.

Torruco-Uco JG, Domínguez-Magaña MA, Dávila-Ortíz G, Martínez-Ayala A, Chel-Guerrero LA, Betancur-Ancona DA. Péptidos antihipertensivos, una alternativa de tratamiento de origen natural: una revisión. *Cienc Tecnol Aliment.* 2008, 6(2):158-168.

Tosh S, Yada S. Dietary fibres in pulse seeds and fractions: characterization, functional attributes, and applications. *Food Res Int.* 2010, 43:450–460.

Traka MH, Spinks CA, Doleman JF, Melchini A, Ball RY, Mills RD, Mithen RF. The dietary isothiocyanate sulforaphane modulates gene expression and alternative gene splicing in a PTEN null preclinical murine model of prostate cancer. *Mol Cancer.* 2010, 9:189.

Utrilla-Coello RG, Osorio-Dcaz P, Bello-Perez L. Alternative use of chickpea flour in bread making: Chemical composition and starch digestibility of bread. *Food Sci Technol Int.* 2007, 13:323-327.

van Breda SG, van Agen E, van Sanden S, Burzykowski T, Kleinjans JC, van Delft JH. Vegetables affect the expression of genes involved in carcinogenic and anticarcinogenic processes in the lungs of female C57Bl/6 mice. *J Nutr.* 2005, 135(11):2546-2552.

van Breda SGJ, van Agen E, van Sanden S, Burzykowski T, Kienhuis AS, Kleinjans JCS, van Delft JHM. Vegetables affect the expression of genes involved in anticarcinogenic processes in the colonic mucosa of C57Bl/6 Female Mice. *J Nutr.* 2005a, 135:1879 – 1888.

Vander Wal JS, Marth JM, Khosla P, Jen KL, Dhurandhar NV. Short-term effect of eggs on satiety in overweight and obese subjects. *J Am Coll Nutr.* 2005, 24:510-515.

Vang O, Rasmussen BF, Andersen O. Combined effects of complex mixtures of potentially anti-carcinogenic compounds on antioxidant enzymes and carcinogen metabolizing enzymes in the rat. *Cancer Lett.* 1997, 114(1–2):283-286.

Vazquez-Prieto MA, Bettaieb A, Haj FG, Fraga CG, Oteiza PI. (-)-Epicatechin prevents TNFα-induced activation of signaling cascades involved in inflammation and insulin sensitivity in 3T3-L1 adipocytes. *Arch Biochem Biophys.* 2012, [Epub ahead of print].

Veldhorst MA, Nieuwenhuizen AG, Hochstenbach-Waelen A, van Vught AJ, Westerterp KR, Engelen MP, Brummer RJM, Deutz NEP, Westerterp-Platenga MS. Dose-dependent satiating effect of whey relative to casein or soy. *Physiol Behav.* 2009, 96:675-682.

Verbeek R, Plomp AC, van Tol EA, van Noort JM: The flavones luteolin and apigenin inhibit *in vitro* antigen-specific proliferation and interferon-gamma production by murine and human autoimmune T cells. *J Altern Complement Med.* 2004, 68:621-629.

Vergara-Castañeda H, Guevara-González R, Guevara-Olvera L, Oomah BD, Reynoso-Camacho R, Wiersma P, Loarca-Piña G. Non-digestible fraction of beans (*Phaseolus vulgaris* L.) modulates signaling pathway genes at an early stage of colon cancer in Sprague–Dawley rats. *Br J Nutr.* 2012, 108:S145–S154.

Vergara-Castañeda HA, Guevara-González RG, Ramos-Gómez M, Reynoso-Camacho R, Guzmán-Maldonado H, Feregrino-Pérez AA, Oomah D, Loarca-Piña G. Non-digestible fraction of cooked bean (*Phaseolus vulgaris* L.) cultivar Bayo Madero suppresses colonic aberrant crypt foci in azoxymethane-induced rats. *Food Funct.* 2010, 1:294–300.

Vermeirssen V, Augustijns P, Morel N, van Camp J, Opsomer A, Verstraete W. *In vitro* intestinal transport and antihypertensive activity of ACE inhibitory pea and whey digests. *Int J Food Sci Nutr.* 2005, 56(6):415-430.

Vioque J, Pedroche J, Yust MM, Lqari H, Megías C, Girón-Calle J, Alaiz M, Millán F. Peptídeos bioativos em proteínas vegetais de reserva. *Braz J Food Technol.* 2006, 51(5):361-365.

Vucenik I, Shamsuddin AM. Protection against cancer by dietary IP6 and inositol. *Nutr Cancer.* 2006, 55:109–125.

Weaver WW. "Peas." *Encyclopedia of Food and Culture.* Ed. Solomon H. Katz. 3 vols. New York: Charles Scribner & Sons, 2003.

Węglarz L, Molin I, Orchel A, Parfiniewicz B, Dzierżewicz Z. Quantitative analysis of the level of *p53* and *p21WAF1* mRNA in human colon cancer HT-29 cells treated with inositol hexaphosphate. *Acta Biochim Pol.* 2006, 53(2):349–356.

Westerterp-Plantenga MS. The significance of protein in food intake and body weight regulation. *Curr Opin Clin Nutr Metab Care,* 2003, 6:635-638.

WHO. 2008. European Action Plan for Food and Nutrition Policy 2007–2012. Available from: http://www.euro.who.int/__data/assets/pdf_file/0017/74402/E91153.pdf

Winham D, Hutchins A. Baked bean consumption reduces serum cholesterol in hypercholesterolemic adults. *Nutr Res.* 2007, 27:380–386.

Woyengo TA, Ramprasath VR, Jones PJH. Anticancer effects of phytosterols. *Eur J Clin Nutr.* 2009, 63:813–820.

Xin L, Yang S Effects of phytic acid on cell cycle and the related protein expression in human hepatoma cell line Hep G2 *in vitro. Acta Nutr Sin.* 2011-05.

Xu B, Chang SK. Phenolic substance characterization and chemical and cell-based antioxidant activities of 11 lentils grown in the northern United States. *J Agric Food Chem.* 2010, 58(3):1509-1517.

Xu BJ, Yuan SH, Chang SKC. Comparative analyses of phenolic composition, antioxidant capacity, and color of cool season legumes and other selected food legumes. *J Food Sci.* 2007, 72(2):S167-S177.

Xu BJ, Yuan SH, Chang SKC. Comparative analyses of phenolic composition, antioxidant capacity, and color of cool season legumes and other selected food legumes. *J Food Sci.* 2007, 72(2):S167-S177.

Xu Q, Kanthasamy AG, Reddy MB. Phytic acid protects against 6-hydroxydopamine-induced dopaminergic neuron apoptosis in normal and iron excess conditions in a cell culture model. *Parkinson's Disease.* 2011,doi:10.4061/2011/431068.

Yamamoto N. Antihypertensive peptides derived from food proteins. *Biopolymers.* 1997, 43:129-134.

Yamsaengsung R, Berghofer E, Schoenlechner R. Physical properties and sensory acceptability of cookies made from chickpea addition to white wheat or whole wheat flour compared to gluten-free amaranth or buckwheat flour. *Int J Food Sci Technology.* 2012, doi: 10.1111/j.1365-2621.2012.03092.x

Yang CS, Chung JY, Yang G, Chhabra SK, Lee MJ. Tea and tea polyphenols in cancer prevention. *J Nutr.* 2000, 130 (2):472S-478S.

Yang Y, Zhou L, Gu Y, Zhang Y, Tang J, Li F, Shang W, Jiang B, Yue X, Chen M. Dietary chickpeas reverse visceral adiposity, dyslipidaemia and insulin resistance in rats induced by a chronic high-fat diet. *Br J Nutr.* 2007, 98(4):720-726.

Ye Y, Hou R, Chen J, Mo L, Zhang J, Huang Y, Mo Z. Formononetin-induced apoptosis of human prostate cancer cells through ERK1/2 mitogen-activated protein kinase inactivation. *Horm Metab Res.* 2012, 44(4):263-267.

Zare F, Champagne CP, Simpsonc BK, Orsata V, Boye JI. Effect of the addition of pulse ingredients to milk on acid production by probiotic and yoghurt starter cultures. *LWT - Food Sci Technology.* 2012, 45(2):155–160.

Zhao QW, Huang X, Lou YJ, Weber N, Proksch P. Effects of ethanol extracts from adzuki bean (*Phaseolus angularis* Wight.) and lima bean (*Phaseolus lunatus* L.) on estrogen and progesterone receptor phenotypes of MCF-7/BOS cells. *Phytother Res.* 2007, 21:648–652.

Zhao YH, Manthey FA, Chang SKC, Hou HJ, Yuan SH. Quality characteristics of spaghetti as affected by green and yellow pea, lentil, and chickpea flours. *J Food Sci.* 2005, 70(6):S371–S376.

Zhou JR, Erdman JW. Phytic acid in health and disease. *Crit Rev Food Sci.* 1995, 35:495–508.

In: Functional Foods
Editors: Aron Robinson and Dominick Emerson
ISBN: 978-1-62417-435-3

Chapter 2

TABLE OLIVES: A NATURAL VEHICLE FOR HEALTH-PROMOTING BACTERIA AND BIOACTIVE COMPOUNDS

C. M. Peres[1], A. Hernandez-Mendonza[1,2], C. Peres[3] and F. X. Malcata[1,4,*]

[1]Instituto de Tecnologia Química e Biológica, Universidade Nova de Lisboa, Avenida da República, Oeiras, Portugal
[2]CIAD – Centro de Investigación en Alimentación y Desarrollo, A. C. Hermosillo, Son., México
[3]INIAV, Avenida da República, EAN, Oeiras, Portugal
[4]Department of Chemical Engineering, University of Porto, Rua Dr. Roberto Frias, Porto, Portugal

ABSTRACT

Available scientific evidence supports claims issued on a few foods (or food components) about their favourable role upon human health – beyond merely responding to basic nutritional requirements. A stronger and stronger consumer awareness has meanwhile shifted to such a tertiary role of foods, especially in view of their efficacy to specifically address chronic diseases and health conditions – including ageing.

Some foods marketed as functional are actually natural whole foods (e.g. plant-based foods, such as fruits, vegetables and whole grains) containing significant amounts of bioactive phytochemicals for which new scientific information was released focusing on their effects upon health; in many instances, functionality of already existing foods needs only be publicized at large. In particular, the fruits of the olive tree (Olea europaea L.) have been for ages consumed as such, or else used as feedstock for oil production; although such a consumption stems solely from nutritional features as part of a regular Mediterranean diet, it has been reported that olive fruits contain 1–3% of their fresh pulp weight of insoluble, or water- and lipid-soluble compounds bearing multiple biological

* Author for correspondence: Tel. (+351) 96 8017411; E-mail: fmalcata@fe.up.pt.

properties – e.g. antioxidant, anticarcinogenic, anti-inflammatory, antimicrobial, antihypertensive, antilipidemic, cardiotonic, laxative and anti-platelet aggregation.

Furthermore, table olives may be considered as effective carriers (and even as a wild source) of lactic acid bacteria bearing probiotic features. Such adventitious strains belong to the Lactobacillus genus – and exhibit a remarkable capacity to tolerate the high acidity and salt content of fermented vegetables, as well as an ability to adhere to the colon wall and survive transit through the gastrointestinal tract. This realization may lead to improvements in the technological aspects of fermentative processing, and as well as emphasize the inherent functional value of fermented table olives – i.e. combine food safety and proactive contribution to human health in a novel manner.

Therefore, this chapter addresses a novel probiotic food by comprehensively and critically reviewing available information on health-promoting phytonutrients and lactic acid bacteria in olives, aiming at a better understanding of its potential toward improvement of health – thus consubstantiating a case study of a plant-based functional food.

1. Introduction

Interest in the relationship between diet, health and well-being has been growing exponentially in Europe, thus mimicking a trend observed also in the rest of the developed world. Foods have indeed been examined intensively for added physiological benefits, including ability to reduce chronic disease risk or otherwise optimize health. Hence, the drive toward functional foods has arisen from the growing consumer interest on the relationship between specific dietary ingredients and health.

Scientists have been rather active in identifying physiologically active components in plants, i.e. phytochemicals that potentially reduce the risk of occurrence of a variety of chronic diseases. In the 1990's, such research efforts unfolded a global interest in functional foods – a term coined to describe foods (or nutrients) that, upon ingestion, lead to physiological changes in the body distinct from those derived from their role as nutrients. An increased awareness of food functionality has paralleled consumer's concerns on life care – as long as they recognize that food can bring about health benefits complementary to traditional medical approaches to treatment of those diseases [1].

A new generation of natural healthy foods has consequently been on the rise – and fermented olives are an excellent example thereof. Recall that concerted policies pertaining to public health aimed at efficiently facing budgetary restrictions require investment on preventive health approaches – especially as human life expectancy is extended; functional foods are seminal vectors towards this strategy [2]. Many technological innovations have meanwhile arisen, driven by realisation of the important role of food in promoting and sustaining health, and the food industry has responded accordingly by redirecting its strategy to foods containing nutraceuticals – i.e. food components with favourable physiological effects upon health [3].

Olive tree (*Olea europaea* L.) belongs to the *Oleaceae* family; it is endemic in dry and temperate regions of the world [4]. This tree is chiefly found in the Mediterranean Basin – which accounts for *ca.* 98% of the world's cultivation [5]. Consumption of olives has increased significantly in recent years – especially in high-income countries, viz. United

States, Europe, Japan, Canada and Australia, thus causing a rapid development of olive-based products [6].

Processed table olives have been available to the general public for generations [7,8]. These foods are consumed as part of a regular diet, and primarily to address basic nutritional purposes. However, several health effects have been investigated – associated with e.g. high contents of monounsaturated fatty acids, vitamins and phenolics, all of which play multiple biological activities. These components also contribute to the unique flavour and taste of olive oil and table olives [9].

Traditionally fermented olives consequently constitute a suitable feedstock for eventual issuing of functional claims; since health sells at high prices and consumers prefer traditional products, innovation should be targeted at identifying other nutraceuticals in said item, and even the possibility of using them as delivery of unusual probiotic strains while keeping its traditional sensory profile.

2. Processing of Table Olives

Olives (mainly from *Olea europea sativa* L.) constitute an important crop in the Mediterranean area with strong historic and economic relevance. Its cultivation probably started *ca.* 6,000 years ago in the region currently called Turkey. Phoenicians introduced it in the Greek islands, from where it expanded to all other Mediterranean countries – where they became an essential element for preservation of ethnicity and environment, to eventually reach a significant weight in national agricultural trades [4]. More recently, this crop was introduced in EUA, South America and Australia [10].

Table olives are an ancient Mediterranean fermented food – a detailed recipe for table olive preparation dates back to 42 a.D.; and as a consequence, the largest consumption also occurs in the major producing countries, with the exception of USA [6]. EU member States contribute with 43.7% to the global table olive production, followed by Arab countries – mainly Turkey, Egypt and Syria. Spain is the main producing country in the world (72.8% of the total EU production), followed by Greece (15.2%) and Italy (9.6%) – whereas the Portuguese table olive production represents a mere 1.6% of the total EU production, and is mostly redirected for internal consumption [6, 11]. Olive fruits have a bitter flavour upon harvest; hence, they typically undergo fermentation, or cure with lye or brine to debitter them and thus make them more palatable. Note that, even when ripe, olives are hardly edible due to astringency [12].

Olive cultivars used for table olive preparation are often of a larger size than those used to manufacture oil. The amount of flesh should not lie below 70% in weight; the oil content should also not be too high to avoid damaging the consistency and hampering preservation of the processed fruit [12, 13]. The fruit grows from July to September-October – when the maximum size is reached. At this time, olives are green – and change their colour gradually, first to straw-yellow, then turning violet and eventually darkening to black. This phenomenon is due to a gradual substitution of chlorophylls by carotenoids – and ends up with accumulation of anthocyanins. According to Romero *et al.* [14], cyanidin 3-rutinoside and 3-glucoside are the most common anthocyanins in fresh ripe olives.

Fermentation is a promising technology toward biopreservation: it not only extends shelf life, but also improves safety at the expense of desirable microorganisms and their metabolites [15]. In table olives, fermentation is also aimed at enhancing the sensory attributes of the final product. A wide diversity of practical recipes, from ancient and local creativity, gave rise to three major processes: Spanish-style green olives in brine, natural black olives in brine and ripe olives darkened by oxidation [12]. As appearance is an important issue to the consumer, harvesting should be manual as much possible to avoid fruit damage [16, 17].

A Spanish-style (pickled) green olives, or treated green olives in brine, refers to a process that involves alkaline treatment prior to brining. The debittering stage is accomplished by immersion of the fruits in a dilute NaOH solution, of 2-3.5% depending on the cultivar, during 6 to 16 hours, until the alkali has diffused *ca.* 2/3 of the whole way through the flesh [7, 10, 13]. The concentration of NaOH, as well as the duration of this treatment affect the permeability of the fruit, but also the medium temperature: dissolution of NaOH in water is in fact higly exothermic, thus facilitating diffusion by also increasing permeability of the fruits via degradation of cell walls, to eventually release the cell contents [13]. Oleuropein and other phenol compounds are hydrolyzed by the alkali, and yield mainly oleoside-11-methylester and hydroxytyrosol – which are unstable in the brine. A lengthy wash is usually carried out, at first with flowing water to remove most NaOH, and then via two or three immersions in fresh water for several hours [7]. This washing step is critical, as some nutrients already decayed and are washed out. It is, nevertheless, important that a portion of NaOH remains in the olive flesh so as to aid in establishment of a buffering capacity afterwards – due chiefly to the conjugated pair lactic acid / sodium lactate [16]. Fruits are then placed in a brine containing NaCl (8-12 %, w/v) and nutrients are allowed to diffuse from the fruit to the brine, while NaCl diffuses into the olives until equilibration. After a few days, NaCl concentration generally stabilises around 5%, so a medium suitable for fermentation has been established. Before shipment, they are placed in a suitable preservation brine containing ca. 5% NaCl (w/v) at pH 4.5 (often adjusted with lactic, citric and acetic acids). A certain level of phenols is expected as it brings about desired sensory features, while assuming an antioxidant capacity for the end product [16].

According to IOOC [10], untreated black olives in brine or plain black olives is a technology applying to fully mature fruits that do not undergo any alkaline treatment. Ripe fruits have softer pulp, richer in sugars and anthocyanins; their high contents in polyaromatic compounds is initially lower than in green olives, yet they can inhibit microbial growth (1.5-2.5%) [10, 13]. Hydroxityrosol was found to be the main phenol compound in ripe olives [18] that are debittered by yeasts and lactic acid bacteria during fermentation.

For the naturally black olives processing (at pH *ca.* 7 or slightly higher), fruits are immersed in brine containing 8-12% NaCl (depending on the country, region and plant); the tissues remain alive, and thus take up nutrients and dissolved O_2 – while releasing CO_2 and heat. Containers are kept full, and tightly closed to avoid growth of oxidative organisms. NaCl is periodically added to the brine so as to maintain its target level of 8% NaCl – to compensate for the amount diffused into the pulp, and to help discriminate the desired microbial population. The pH usually decreases to reach *ca.* 4; the end of the process is indicated by brine turning clear, as bacterial growth stops due to nutrient depletion thus causing cell sedimentation. Fruits also tend to lie on the bottom of the container due to brine absorption. Colour and acidity corrections are sometimes implemented via air oxidation and acid addition, respectively [16]. The composition of the brine varies according to local traditions; often times, olive oil, vinegar and spices are added, as well as authorized preservatives [10].

In the Californian method, or ripe olives darkened by oxidation, no fermentation takes place – or is irrelevant for the characteristics of the final product. The olives undergo sequential lye treatments using 1-2% NaOH that penetrates the fruit to the pit; at the end of each treatment, olives are washed with water and aerated for some time. Alkaline oxidization causes gradual darkening of the fruit, but dramatically changes its texture. Colour changes of the olive flesh are due to oxidation and polymerization of phenolic compounds [13], particularly anthocyanins [14]. This process entails a substantial removal of phenol compounds by alkaline hydrolysis [13] with the black colour being stabilized with ferrous gluconate or lactate. Olives are finally canned in the brine, and subjected to heat treatment to further extend their shelf life [16].

Fermented foods constitute in general an important ingredient of the human diet in many developing countries; although fermentation has been used for thousands of years for preservation (and even improvement) of foods, the underlying microbial and enzymatic processes are still largely unknown. In the particular case of olive fermentation, artisanal processes are associated with a rather wide microbial strain diversity – especially in small artisanal units, which also causes fluctuations in final product quality. Conversely, industrial plants resort to simpler and more standard manufacture methods, so the final product bears a more constant quality level and homogenous features. Note that use of starters minimizes the risk of product spoilage, but also constrains strain biodiversity [19]. Fermentations are typically carried out by bacteria and yeasts, and are aimed at facilitating preservation and storage; they also serve to reduce generation of detrimental components, and improve nutritional and health features in food products [20, 21], as well as for production of physiologically beneficial components, *e.g.* via increasing the levels of antioxidants [22].

Natural fermentation and green Spanish style rely on spontaneous fermentation carried out by epiphytic microbiota (mainly yeasts and lactic acid bacteria); the optimum fermentation temperature is 24 ^{0}C, and the process usually takes place for 2-3 months. Once fermentation is complete, olives are packed in air-tight jars – and may undergo heat-sterilization afterwards to obtain a more stable product [16]. The fermentation process of green olives usually starts with Gram-negative bacteria, which after a week are expected to vanish. At pH below 6, lactobacilli develop massively – as Gram-negative bacteria are depleted and the brine attains a pH of 4.5 [7]. Homolactic strains of *Lactobacillus plantarum* and *Lactobacillus pentosus* have been found, in standard fermentations, while nutrients remain; at low carbohydrate levels, acid formation slows down and so do the numbers of viable yeasts accompanying the lactobacilli [8, 10, 23]: yeasts degrade phenol compounds, and supply vitamins and amino acids required by lactobacilli [24]. In this type of association, the microbiota change their individual metabolic pathways – and the unique metabolites they accumulate will strongly contribute to the final aroma of olives [25].

In the first stages of fermentation, microbial growth appears to compete with plant tissues for nutrients – as the latter are still respiring, and thus consuming dissolved O_2 and cellular reserves. The predominant family until the second week is *Enterobacteriaceae* [7, 26]; they produce organic acids, ethanol, CO_2 and H_2. At this stage, it is necessary to keep the NaCl level above 8-10% to favour dominance of yeasts, particularly *Torulaspora delbrueckii*, *Debaryomyces hansenii* and *Cryptococcus laurentii* [26, 27]. In Portuguese olive fermentation, the yeast population has been found to include *Pichia membranaefaciens*, *Pichia fermentans*, *Saccharomyces cerevisiae* and *Candida oleophila*, all of which appear to exhibit desirable technological features including synthesis of B-complex vitamins [24]; this has been confirmed in Spanish fermentation [28]. Furthermore, antimicrobial activity against selected food-borne bacterial pathogens was observed, as well as release of mycotoxins. *Pichia membranaefaciens* and *C. oleophila* are likelly the best candidates for eventual inclusion in tailor-made probiotic starter/adjunct cultures [24, 29]. Yeasts are apparently responsible for fermentation in the first weeks in brines; during this stage, pH drops to 4.5-4.8, and the predominant population is made up of yeast species and members of the *Lactobacillus*, *Leuconostoc* and *Pediococcus* bacterial genera [16, 27]. As before, homolactic strains of *L. plantarum* and *L. pentosus* have been recorded in standard fermentations, together with yeasts [8]. Both play an important role in biological debittering, since some strains can degrade oleuropein [30, 31]. This fermentation process is longer than in the Sevillian style preparation, thus leading to a slightly more bitter and less acidic final product. According to Garrido-Fernández *et al.* [16], pH should stabilise between 5.5 and 4.5, corresponding to 0.3 to 0.5% w/v of lactic acid in brine.

Main causes for table olive recall are associated with incorrect fermentations; for instance, the initial populations are of a Gram-negative nature that is often associated with hygienic issues,, and their growth is favoured by NaCl concentrations below 7% – they cause sloughing, abnormal colorations and off-flavours. Excessive aerobic conditions may favour development of oxidative yeasts inside the flesh, thus forming gas pockets or fish eyes. Establishment of correct homolactic fermentation, at later stages, prevents growth of spoilage yeasts. On the other hand, abnormal fermentations, *e.g.* associated with putrid and butyric flavours, occur upon establishment of populations of *Clostridium* and *Propionibacterium* sp. [7, 16]. An increase in pH and volatile acidity accompanies these changes, thus opening the way for growth of other undesirable microorganisms. In the case of naturally black olives, fungi readily adapt to the prevailing environmental conditions at the initial stages, but their development should be avoided via anaerobiosis – *e.g.* by keeping containers totally full. Moulds may rise pH and soften olive pulp through pectinolytic enzymes; in addition, some species release toxins [16].

As emphasized above, *Lactobacillus* sp. are the main responsible for extension of the shelf life of table olives, as a direct (or indirect) consequence of accumulation of primary metabolites (*e.g.* lactic acid), bacteriocins (i.e. anti-microbial peptides) and other anti-oxidizing compounds that inhibit undesirable microorganisms and degradation reactions. Bacteriocin-producers readily establish in standard fermentations, and have thus attracted a great interest from the food industry – aiming, in particular, at their potential toward food preservation. One bacteriocin, plantaricin S, seems to be widely widespread in these environments – and it is quite common in Spanish olives [32], as well as in Portuguese table-olives. The corresponding operon can be found – sometimes with slight sequence variations, even in multiple bacteriocin producers. Bacteriocin production throughout fermentation can be enhanced by adjusting selected technological factors [33, 34]. Despite their usefulness, further studies are needed to better clarify the role of bacteriocins in controlling certain populations – as well as their relation to factors inherent to the 'terroir' and olive variety. As specific microorganisms account for specific flavour notes, a better knowledge on the microecology of good quality table olives is missing. Once such aspects are clarified, some of these strains could be used as starters – thus reducing fluctuations in quality level, while permitting reliable scale-up.

Novel applications for lactic bacteriocins have also received the attention of several authors. According to WHO [35], *ca.* 70% of bacteria that cause infections in hospitals are resistant to, at least, one of the drugs most commonly used to treat infections (i.e. antibiotics). Since bacteriocin-resistance mechanisms are distinct from those of antibiotics – and are not genetically transferred, they may constitute a suitable alternative, or at least a complement to common antibiotics in treating pathogenic strains exhibiting multiple antibiotic resistances [36].

An ecosystem that has also received an increasing interest is the gastrointestinal tract, especially with regard to inclusion of probiotic lactobacilli in the diet – as they are frequently associated with bacteriocin production. Many commercial probiotics belong to *L. plantarum* – which is a very common species in fermented olives; this bacterium withstands the harsh conditions prevailing during gastric and intestinal digestion. Such probiotics may, in combination with antibiotics, increase the rate of eradication and/or decrease adverse effects of the classical approach to eradication of *Helicobacter pylori* [37-39].

3. High-Value Nutrients and Functional Compounds of Table Olives

Table olives constitute a highly nutritive and balanced food, yet they entertain a poor bad image owing to high contents of fat and salt. To circumvent these myths, table olive has been promoted as healthy food supported on a number of studies (*e.g.* [40]).

The distribution and structure of the chemical constituents of olive fruit is complex, and depends on such parameters as cultivar, cultivation practices, geographical origin and level of maturation. On average, the pericarp includes water (70-75%), protein (1.6%), oil (15-30%), carbohydrate (19.1%), cellulose (5.8%), inorganic substances (1.5%), phenolic compounds (1–3%), pectin, organic acids, vitamins and pigments [5, 7]. Organic acids appear as intermediate products of degradation of other compounds [41]. Of particular relevance is the high content in dietary fibers and vitamins (especially carotenes, tocopherols and thiamine), regardless of some differences in cultivar composition [40].

The oil content increases during maturation and depends chiefly on the cultivar. It consists mainly of two components, saponifiables (*ca.* 98%) comprising triacylglycerols, partial glycerides, esters of fatty acids or free fatty acids, and phosphatides; and unsaponifiables (1–2%) – mainly minor components, *e.g.* tocopherols, phytosterols, pigments and phenolics [42].

Triacylglycerols are triesters of glycerol; the most abundant combination in olive oil is oleic-oleic-oleic (OOO), followed (by order of incidence) by palmitic-oleic-oleic (POO), oleic-oleic-linoleic (OOL), palmitic-oleic-linoleic (POL) and stearic-oleic-oleic (SOO) [43]. Such triglycerides are chiefly accounted for by monounsaturates (*ca.* 80%), e.g. oleic acid, along with small amounts of saturates and considerable quantity of polyunsaturates possessing 18 carbon atoms (C18) – which are fatty acids essential for human nutrition, *e.g.*

linoleic (18:2, ω-6) and α-linolenic (18:3, ω-3) [44]. These fatty acids are indeed indispensable to cell structure development and function, but cannot be synthesized by the human body [40].

Phytosterols include a major proportion of unsaponifiables, are biosynthetically derived from squalene – and may represent up to 90% of these compounds, at concentrations of 1250-7500 mg kg^{-1}; they entail a group of triterpenes, the content of which ranges from 1000 to 2300 ppm. Squalene is followed by carotenoids; β-carotene – the precursor of vitamin A, is the most abundant (0.9 to 5.0 mg kg^{-1}). Also present are lycopene and other linear (or branched) hydrocarbons, some of which have been found in the volatile fraction (viz. phenanthrene, anthracene and pyrene) at trace levels [45].

The sterol esters, *ca.* 2600 mg kg^{-1}, are also important compounds within the aforentioned group – mainly sitosterol, campesterol and stigmasterol; their profile is a form of fingerprint, and may thus be used to classify olive oils from distinct regions. From a nutritional point of view, the most common is β-sitosterol (ca. 90%) that helps reduce absorption of cholesterol [46]. Tocopherols (α-, β-, γ- and δ-tocopherol), at ratios of 150-200 mg kg^{-1} in olive oil, are considered as the most important lipid-soluble natural antioxidants, and are able to prevent lipid peroxidation and participate in the structure of vitamin E. They are thermolabile, so they vanish during the refining process [47].

Table olives supply *ca.* 250 kcal/100 g – i.e. less than half what is normally found in chips (560 kcal) or dark chocolate (534 kcal). According to Garrido-Fernández and Lopez-Lopez [40], olives are an important dietary source of fiber (2-3%) that determines texture and digestibility of the olive fruit as a whole [48]. The levels of vitamins in the olive pulp are also important; the dominant are (water-soluble) ascorbic acid (vitamin C) and thiamine (vitamin B_1), and (oil-soluble) tocopherols (vitamin E) and carotenes (pro-vitamin A). Olives contain also small amounts of lutein and zeaxanthin, which are antioxidant compounds closely related to vitamin A [49]. In the traditional Spanish-style green olive fermentation, the four vitamins essential to growth of *L. plantarum* are required: nicotinic and pantothenic acids, biotin and vitamin B6 are indeed available in the fermentation brines within the first few days of processing, but their levels throughout the fermentative process usually lie well above said microbial requirements [28, 50].

Various yeast strains isolated from brines were reported to hold a metabolism leading to synthesis of essential growth factors for lactobacilli, *e.g.* vitamins – so at early stages of fermentation, yeasts appear to play a symbiotic role encompassing *L. plantarum* [24, 51].

The mineral composition of table olives depends on both cultivar and preparation style. As expected for a brined food product, Na is the most abundant element – but olives are also a good source of Ca, K, Mg and P. The concentration of Fe is high in ripe olives, but relatively low in green and directly brined ones – whereas the microelements Cu, Zn, Se and Mn are found at levels similar to those in other plants [7].

Processing affects the mineral content (except Ca and Mg) of table olives between green (Spanish style), directly brined and ripe olives; the most discriminating elements appears to be Fe, K, Na, Mn, Cu and P (between styles), and these plus Mg and Ca (between cultivars) [52].

Phenolic compounds are well-known secondary metabolites that can be synthesized by plants in response to stress conditions [53]. They contribute towards the sensory characteristics of olive products, but impart also pharmaceutical and physiological benefits

[13, 54]. The phenolic profile in olives is very complex, and the average concentration of such compounds (40-900 mg kg^{-1}) depends on several factors including cultivar, environment and processing technology [14, 55, 56]. The main classes of phenolics in olive oil are phenolic acids, phenolic alcohols, hydroxy-isocromans, flavonoids, secoiridoids and lignans [57, 58]. Several phenolic acids, *e.g.* gallic, protocatechuic, *p*-hydroxybenzoic, vanillic, caffeic, syringic, *p*- and *o*-coumaric, ferulic acid, and cinnamic acids have been determined in olive oil. Phenolic acids are, together with phenyl-alcohols, hydroxy-isochromans and flavonoids, present in small amounts, whereas secoiridoids and lignans dominate within this family of compounds [59]. The main hydroxycinnamic acid derivative in olive fruit is verbascoside. Secoiridoids are derivatives of oleuropein, demethyloleuropein and ligstroside [59, 60]. The antioxidant properties of olives are due to free phenolics and their glycosides, which constitute 1-3% of pulp wet weight. The most relevant in the oil fraction are anthocyanins, while oleuropein dominates in the aqueous fraction [13].

Oleuropein is the main responsible for bitterness of olive fruits; its content is higher at the first stages of maturation, and in green cultivars than in black olives, whereas anthocyanins tend to increase along maturation. The reduction in oleuropein level is accompanied by an increase in the levels of its glycosylated secondary products – which reach maximum values in black olives [61]. Recall that oleuropein is the ester between 2-(30, 40-dihydroxyphenyl) ethanol (hydroxytyrosol) and the oleosidic skeleton common to the glycosidic secoiridoids of typical Oleaceae [62]. Oleuropein is degraded during fermentation, thus leading to accumulation of derivatives with higher antioxidant capacity such as hydroxytyrosol. Hydroxytyrosol appears as a simple or esterified phenol (with elenoic acid), thus forming oleuropein or its aglycone, but also as part of the verbascoside molecule [61]; the content in such antioxidant phenolic compounds is noteworthy when compared to other fruits. Pereira *et al.* [63] claimed that the phenol content of Portuguese table olives could be as high as 5 g kg^{-1} of fruit, in the case of naturally black or Sevillian style; the phenolic fraction contains mostly hydroxytyrosol, besides relevant amounts of tyrosol, luteonin and α-tocopherol. Flavonoids such as luteolin and apigenin were also reported in olives [64] – and lignans have been recently isolated and characterized [65].

4. Biological Activities and Health Benefits of Table Olives

The Mediterranean diet is a good example of low saturated fat-rich diets that can be replaced in attempts to find a healthy model to be recommended. Owing to its nuclear status in this diet, and thanks to extensive research on its unique phytonutrient composition, olives and olive oil have become a classical culinary ingredient with very difficult-to-match health benefits [66]. A lower prevalence of non-communicable diseases, such as cardiovascular diseases and certain types of cancers, has in fact been demonstrated in Mediterranean countries, and claimed to be directly related to consumption of olive oil and other components of the Mediterranean diet [67].

The health-related properties of table olives are similar to those of olive oil, as expected; health-protective nutrients have been identified in olives, and recent studies have taken a closer look at olive cultivars and processing, and changes undergone ly olive nutrients. As one ages, the digestive capacity markedly reduces, thus resulting in harder absorption nutrients from food – especially vitamins and minerals. Since olive products are very digestible, its nutrients aid in digestion and stimulate appetite. Given olive nutrient richness, it is not surprising that a larger and larger set of documented health benefits exists encompassing most body systems [68].

Several public-health based studies have accordingly revealed that olives and olive oil are strongly linked to a lower prevalence of cardiovascular diseases [54, 69] and certain cancers [70, 71]. Several beneficial aspects, *e.g.* vasodilator capacity, anti-platelet aggregation [72], anti-inflammatory (*e.g.* arthritis and asthma) [73], antioxidant [74] and antimicrobial [75-77], as well as in immune system stimulation have been associated to the high iron content [78, 79].

Olives are also the best fruit source of (trace) copper; this element helps the body absorb the iron present in olives, thus reducing tissue damage arising from free radicals; it also assists in formation of muscle fibres and strong bones, protects connective tissues, preserves myelin sheath of nerves, enhances melanin production, and assists thyroid gland functioning. Note that higher levels of energy are produced as more enzymes are synthetized in the presence of high iron levels [80].

Copper and iron are minerals essential also for a healthy blood. The high iron content of olives facilitates formation of hemoglobin in red blood cells that are the carriers of oxygen in the body. Calcium is also abundant in olives and is necessary for a smooth functioning of heart muscles, transmission of nerve impulses, muscle growth and blood clotting, besides enzyme activity optimization. In addition, olives contain magnesium and phosphorus – which, together with calcium, are the three essentials minerals for a healthy heart; and zinc, which is essential in the digestion process and in the control of insulin – besides being required for DNA and protein synthesis, immune support and wound healing, as well as alcohol breakdown [81].

Dietary fibre is classically defined as the total polysaccharide and lignin fraction of the diet that is not digested by endogenous secretions in the digestive tract [82]. Olives are among the fruits with an appreciable content of dietary fibre, arising from biochemical changes of the cell wall polysaccharides during ripening and postharvest processing; recent studies point at the beneficial effects upon prevention of a few human pathologies relating to digestion, as well as cholesterol-lowering [83].

While commonly recognized as a high-fat food (80-85% of the calories in olives do indeed come from fat), olives contain more (monoinsaturated) oleic acid and less (polyunsaturated) linoleic and linolenic acids than other vegetable oils. They provide almost ¾ of their fat as oleic acid, and smaller amounts of the essential fatty linoleic acid, and an even smaller amounts of α-linolenic acid – as well as of Ω-3 fatty acids, the levels of which change throughout ripening [84]. During olive fermentation, lipase and esterase activities in yeast increase the free fatty acid level in brines [85], thus leading to different fatty acid composition and fat content of various commercial table olives [86].

When diets low in monounsaturated fat are altered via increases in monounsaturated fat content (without changing the total fat), a decrease in the blood cholesterol ratio (high density lipoprotein, HDL, cholesterol to low density lipoprotein, LDL, cholesterol) was experienced by human volunteers [87]. Oleic acid can prevent cardiovascular diseases – which are the major cause of mortality in industrialized countries [88], by increasing plasma HDL cholesterol and apoprotein A1, and decreasing LDL cholesterol and apoprotein B [87]. The consumption of saturated fatty acids should in fact be moderate, and approximately equal to the intake of polyunsaturated ones; a balanced lipid intake should entail a total amount of fats of 25 to 30% of the total calories, with proportions in fatty acids of 6–8% monounsaturated, 12–14% polyunsaturated as ω-6, and 0.5–1.5% polyunsaturated as ω-3 [42]. Medical studies have indicated that diets deficient in vitamin E accelerate degradation of certain fatty acids – in a process invariably associated with age. The vitamin E content in olive is in fact thought to provide a defence against such effects, and is useful to help maintain mental capacities and muscule control; it has also been shown to improve T cell function in the older, through a significant impact upon expression of genes associated with them [89].

In addition to the large amount of monounsaturated fatty acids, the nutritional value and health functions of olive products are ascribed also to such minor components as aliphatic and triterpenic alcohols, sterols (mainly β-sitosterol), hydrocarbons (squalene), volatile compounds, tocopherols (chiefly α-tocopherol), pigments (e.g. chlorophylls), carotenoids (β-carotene and lutein) and antioxidants [56, 90]. The modes of action are actually related to two underlying health-support aspects of olives: their unique antioxidant [66] and anti-inflammatory features, namely via inflammatory mediator production by human mononuclear cells [91].

Triterpenic acids are widespread in plants – in the form of free acids or aglycones for triterpenoid saponins. Among the free triterpenic acids, oleanolic and maslinic are probably the most abundant in plants – and olive fruits and leaves are especially rich therein. Based on their structural characteristics, their effect on biophysical properties of cell membranes has been claimed to play a biological role [92]. Because of a recent interest on triterpenic acids of olives, a deeper knowledge of their contents in commercial table olives, and a better understanding of their changes during processing is in order. Differences were found between cultivars and processing technologies; for instance, Hojiblanca has a higher amount of triterpenic acids than Manzanilla cultivars. The concentration of triterpenic acids in commercial table olives is more affected by the alkaline treatment and extra washing cycles than other variables [93].

Results by Juan *et al.* [94] confirmed inhibition of cell proliferation (without cytotoxicity) and restoration of apoptosis sensitivity in human HT29 colon cancer cells, via the intrinsic mitochondrial pathway, brought about by maslinic and oleanolic acids in olive fruit extracts; this suggests a novel therapeutic strategy for treatment of colon carcinoma [95]. Maslinic acid also hinders spreading of HIV by inhibiting the action of a (serine) protease that uses the virus to burst the cell walls prior to establishment [96]. Maslistic acid also inhibits development of some Apicomplexan species, including *Eimeria, Toxoplasma* and *Neospora,* at multiple intraerythrocytic stages of the parasite; depending on the dose and incubation time, it behaves as a plasmodial parasitostatic compound with a potential therapeutic interest [97].

Human and animal studies have shown that phenolic compounds in olive oil possess important biological activities that may prevent evolution of chronic degenerative diseases. Epidemiological studies have unfolded a relationship between consumption of phenolic-rich foods or beverages and prevention of diseases resulting from oxidative stress – which leads to formation of reactive oxygen species responsible for development of diseases targeting lipids, proteins and deoxyribonucleic acid in living organisms. Some data have pointed at favourable effects upon thrombosis, and tumor genesis and promotion [98]. Phenolic compounds originated in olives have good bioavailability in humans, even at small doses (22 g d^{-1}) – which is lower than those reported in the Mediterranean diet (30–50 g d^{-1}) [99].

During olive fermentation, lipase and β-glucosidase yeast activity increased the concentration of several antioxidant compounds; *P. anomala* exhibited the highest antioxidant capacity in *in vitro* assays [50]. Said enzymatic ability was confirmed in lactic acid bacteria from olive brines [100]: the resulting compounds, particularly hydroxytyrosol, have been claimed to protect against chronic and degenerative diseases better than unsaturated fatty acids themselves [101].

The therapeutic potential of antioxidant compounds relates to their radical-scavenging ability – they can break chain reactions triggered by free radicals [102]. Consequently, they avoid activation of platelet-derived growth factor receptors, and thus formation of amyloidal plaques, inflammation and formation of peroxynitrites – the main cause of memory impairment in Alzheimer's disease; they also contribute to increase acetylcholine as critical compound for short-term memory. Oleocanthal has been implicated in a reduced incidence of Alzheimer’s disease in Mediterranean populations via two mechanisms. Note that in Alzheimer’s disease, a microtubule-associated protein (Tau), involved in promotion of microtubule assembly and stability, begins to aggregate into neurofibrillary tangles [103]; Pitt *et al.* [104] demonstrated that oleocanthal inhibits Tau aggregation. β-amyloidal (Aβ) oligomers (also referred to as ADDLs) have also been suggested as involved in development of Alzheimer’s disease, by protecting neurons from ADDL-induced synaptic deterioration; additionally, they promote antibody clearance of ADDLs [105].

Oxidative stress leads to the onset of atherosclerosis, by inducing lipid peroxidation; antioxidants can prevent it by oxidative modification of LDL [106]. Epidemiological studies have claimed a direct correlation between the Mediterranean diet and a lower incidence of cardiovascular diseases, thus proving that the phenolic compounds of extra-virgin olive oil are a key factor in pathogenesis of atherosclerosis damage through inhibition of LDL oxidation [62, 107].

The reduction in oleuropein levels during fermentation is accompanied by an increase in the levels of its glycosylated secondary products, *e.g.* tyrosol and hydroxytyrosol [60, 99]; this metabolic phenomenon is due to esterase and β-glucosidase activities from lactic acid bacteria and yeasts [2, 24]. Besides phenol compound degradation, olive fermentation plays an important role in inhibition of lipid peroxidation [108]. Hydroxytyrosol appears to be safe, so it has been recognized as GRAS – and future use as human diet supplement is likely. Based on their ability to inhibit formation of peroxides, it has been shown that hydroxytyrosol, and caffeic and protocatechuic acids have a particularly high protective activity [109]. Hydroxytyrosol helps protect cells lining the blood vessels from damage by highly reactive oxygen molecules [110]. While most studies in this area were conducted in laboratory animals, better levels of calcium in the blood have repeatedly been associated with olive oil intake [111].

The bacteriostatic and bacteriocidal activities of oleuropein, as well as hydroxytyrosol and tyrosol derived therefrom have been studied *in vitro* towards many pathogenic bacteria, fungi, viruses and protozoa. Those compounds are able to inhibit production of enterotoxin B by *Staphylococcus aureus*, development of *Salmonella enteritidis* and germination of spores of *Bacillus cereus* [112, 113]. Hydroxytyrosol is highly toxic to *Pseudomonas syringae* pv. *savastanoi* and *Corynebacterium michiganense* – being both phytopathogens; and tyrosol may act as a mycotoxin [114]. Oleuropein can also interfere with synthesis of the amino acids necessary for viral activity – thus preventing diffusion, development and attack on the cell membrane; it also inhibits reproduction and, in the case of retroviruses, synthesis of reverse transcriptase and protease. Finally, oleuropein stimulates phagocytic response of the immune system against pathogenic microorganisms [115]. A bactericidal effect has been observed upon a wide range of bacteria, but not on yeasts [24]; however, oleuropein plays a role (though only slight) upon delaying development and sporulation of *Aspergillus parasiticus*, and production of aflatoxin is notably reduced as well [116]. The effective destruction of microorganisms indicates that olive phenolics may be a useful therapeutic agent in treatment of selected infectious diseases [62].

Hydroxytyrosol also has a potential in preventing bone loss [117]; Several recent laboratory animal studies have found increased depositing of calcium in bone, and decreased loss of total bone mass following consumption of this olive phytonutrient together with oleuropein [118]. That oil present in olives may also have special bone benefits for post-menopausal women, since improved blood markers of overall bone health were found in female rats fed with olive oil after their ovaries had been removed [119].

A diet rich in olive oil is apparently able to protect from mental illness; evidence gathered revealed that volunteers, following a high intake of a hydrogenated fat found mainly in processed foods, experienced up to 48% higher risk of depression compared to volunteers who did not consume such fats – in a dose-response relationship. Cardiovascular disease and depression may indeed share some common mechanisms related to the diet – and a Mediterranean diet rich in olives (besides vegetables, beans and fruits) was actually claimed to make it 30% less likely for one to suffer from depression [120]; this corroborates realization of a greater incidence of depression in countries of Northern of Europe as compared to Southern Europe, which may be due to the Mediterranean diet of the latter.

The phenolic constituents of olives have been associated with potent biological activities *in vitro* besides antioxidant action; tyrosol and hydroxytyrosol are absorbed by humans after ingestion in a dose-dependent manner, and excreted in the urine as glucuronide conjugates [121] – and an increase in the dose of phenolics administered apparently increases the proportion of conjugation with glucuronide [122]. The beneficial effects of the phenolic compounds in olives upon blood pressure apparently derive from their protective effect upon the vascular endothelial function and the presence of calcium antagonists [123].

Phenolic compounds display also a number of pharmacological properties in the gut – where they act as antisecretory, cytoprotective and antioxidant agents; they have also been highligted for their anti-ulcerogenic activity, with a good level of gastric protection, thus constituting an alternative for treatment of gastric ulcers. Antitumor effects of olive constituents have been reported for such organs of the body as pancreas, oral cavity, oesophagus, colon-rectum, prostate and lung; amphiphilic phenolics possess, in fact, the ability to modulate enzymes involved in key functions of those cells [117, 124].

Flavonoids have been reported to act in the gastrointestinal tract via antispasmodic [125], anti-secretory, antidiarraeal [126] and antiulcer [127] mechanisms; the underlying biological effects have been attributed to their antioxidant properties, such as the ability to scavenge free radicals, break radical chain reactions, reduce peroxides and stimulate the enzyme activities of antioxidative defence.

Tannins prevent ulcer development due to their protein-precipitating and vasoconstricting effects – which are also responsible for their astringency. They form a layer over the lining that hinders induced gastric ulcer in rats, while protecting the underlying mucosa from reduction in ulcer scores [127]. The mechanisms of protection of the mucosa against a variety of ulcerogenic agents consequently appear to be mainly free-radical scavenging, increased mucus production, antisecretory action and inhibition of *Helicobacter pylori* growth [128]. Hence, future antiulcer drugs may take advantage of said olive compounds [129].

Hydroxytyrosol was found to considerably inhibit chemically-induced platelet aggregation *in vitro*, accumulation of (pro-aggregating) thromboxane in human serum, production of (pro-inflammatory) leukotrienes by activated human leukocytes, and inhibition of arachidonate lipoxygenase activity [130]. In particular, hydroxytyrosol and oleuropein scavenge superoxide, and thus inhibit platelet aggregation while potentiating nitric oxide-mediated macrophagic immune response [72].

Hydroxytyrosol and related olive phenols have been tested, as supplements, in humans – and it can retain the antioxidant activity following ingestion; the human metabolic pathway has been elucidated, and suggests extensive glucuronidation and subsequent urinary excretion – with a protective role from second hand smoke-induced oxidative damage, inhibition of platelet aggregation, and increases of brain cell resistance to oxidation and mitochondrial membrane potential [99]. Further experiments have confirmed the anti-thrombotic potential of hydroxytyrosol, coupled with its ability to ameliorate osteoarthritis [131].

Obesity has constituted an epidemic burden in modern countries, and has consequently urged public health strategies toward dietary models that can reduce its incidence – and the related metabolic syndrome of diabetes, both of which are characterized by a high cardiovascular risk. Evidence that phenolic compounds play active roles against obesity has appeared more and more often in the scientific literature – including *in vitro* and *in vivo* effects upon induction of pre-adipocytic and adipocytic apoptosis, and inhibition of adipocytic lipid accumulation [132]. New insights of olive oil effects upon obesity have unfolded cardiac metabolic changes, thus demonstrating (for the first time) that olive oil enhances fat oxidation and regulates myocardial metabolic enzymes that may eventually optimize cardiac energy metabolism [133].

5. Fermentation of Table Olives

The fermentation of brined vegetables has traditionally depended on growth of a complex dynamic microbiota, able to metabolize substrates therein (*e.g.* glucose, fructose and mannitol) to organic acids; together with added salt (4-12%), this leads to a preservation effect, as well as improvement of palatability [134].

The spontaneous fermentations observed in different table olive processes are usually the result of competitive activities of the native microbiota that involves the action of homo- and hetero-fermentative lactic acid bacteria (LAB) and/or yeasts; this depends on the cultivar itself, and on the prevailing agricultural and industrial practices. During normal conditions of fermentation, lactic and acetic acids are produced that increase the acidity level of the brine, and lower its pH to 3.8-4.2 [135].

In general, microbial growth during natural fermentation of olives has been categorized into three different stages. Gram-negative bacteria, mainly belonging to the *Enterobacteriaceae* family, appear during initiation. These bacteria decrease in the second stage (primary fermentation), being inhibited by the gradual growth of LAB belonging to *Leuconostoc* and *Pediococcus* genera. The third stage (secondary fermentation) is characterized by proliferations of several strong homofermentative species of lactobacilli. A few yeast species coexist with LAB throughout the entire process of olive brining [24, 136, 137].

The main LAB genus isolated in table olives is *Lactobacillus*, being *Lactobacillus plantarum, Lactobacillus pentosus* and *Lactobacillus paraplantarum* (to a lesser extent) the predominant species – although differences in olive cultivar, geographical origin and processing method can modulate the microecology, including growth of such other lactobacilli as *Lactobacillus casei, Lactobacillus paracasei* and *Lactobacillus brevis,* or of *Enterococcus, Pediococcus, Leuconostoc* and *Lactococcus* spp. [100, 137-141].

Several intrinsic factors – *e.g.* indigenous microbial association and spatial distribution of microorganisms on the olive, pH, water activity, availability of nutrients diffusing from the tissue, structure of the olive skin, and levels of inherent antimicrobial compounds (such as oleuropein and organic acids); and extrinsic factors – *e.g.* temperature, residual NaOH and washing process, oxygen availability, salt concentration, and size and type of fermentation vats, can influence the metabolism of bacteria – and thus the progress of fermentation [141-143]. To improve fermentation and produce consistent and high-quality final products, strict process control of the above intrinsic and extrinsic factors has been recommended – e.g. resorting to starter cultures.

Other factors have provided an additional motivation for use of starter cultures. The large volumes of high salty brines generated by olive fermentation raise significant environmental problems; physicochemical treatments of those wastewaters can reduce up to 75-85% the organic contaminants, yet chlorides remain in solution and still represent a major concern. Salt-free fermentation would be the most obvious solution; nevertheless, salt provides an effective means to control the microbiota, so conducting a natural fermentation at low-salt concentrations will hardly be satisfactory. Conversely, less salt could be used if the background flora was controlled otherwise – and a starter culture based on specific acid lactic bacteria may be a solution to handle the environment and aid in control of fermentation itself [144].

In a controlled fermentation, selected bacteria are added as (single or mixed) starter cultures, mainly to degrade oleuropein and thus avoid bitterness – as well as to reduce the metabolic energy required by the process, and to produce desirable acids and alcohols, with several organoleptic and nutritional advantages associated [145]. Therefore, strain selection is necessary – and should be based on the olive cultivar and processing method at stake (Table 1).

The microorganisms (either as single inoculum or co-culture) currently available – or likely to be considered for use as starter cultures, include many of the species ordinarily isolated from olive fermentations, *e.g. L. plantarum* [19, 146], *L. pentosus* [147, 148], *Leuconostoc cremoris and Leuconostoc paramesenteroides* [149], and *L. brevis* and *L. paracasei* [140].

Table 1. Selection criteria for table olive fermentation

Fast and predominant growth
Homofermentative metabolism
High acidification rate and fast consumption of fermentable substrates
Salt, organic acid and medium polyphenol tolerance
Minimum nutritional requirements
Flavor development
Temperature range for growth
Oleuropein-splitting capacity
Antimicrobial compound production
Bacteriophage resistance
Non-pectinolytic
Unable to produce dextrans or other polysaccharides
Unable to produce biogenic amines

(adapted from [135, 141, 145]).

The specific technological traits thought to be advantageous were assessed in the case of *L. pentosus* CECT 5138 upon inoculation at alkaline pH on lye-treated green olives [150]. Results indicated that cultures grew and underwent accelerated fermentation, thus suggesting a feasible utilization of green olives for inoculation without requiring previous pH correction, or deliberately brought about by other microorganisms. Another study attempted to determine the effects of *L. plantarum* strain LAB B1-2001 on the fermentation of naturally green olives following the traditional Greek method; the starter culture shortened the processing time for preparation of naturally green olives, and positively affected fermentation and acidification rate. Furthermore, olives fermented with LAB B1-2001 were perceived by panellists as less bitter and more aromatic than those fermented spontaneously [146].

A noticeable β-glucosidase activity of *L. plantarum* has been observed that contributes to the olive debittering process [151]; this feature has been found also in *L. pentosus*, *L. brevis* and *Pediococcus pentosaceus* [100]. Another important trait of starter cultures is their ability to grow at low temperature: Kumral *et al.* [149] demonstrated that use of *L. brevis*, *L. cremoris* and/or *L. paramesenteroides* as starters permitted naturally black olive (Gemlik cultivar) processing to be carried out at 10-12 °C and a salt concentration of 7%.

On the other hand, olives can tolerate a modest heat treatment – but thermal inactivation of undesired microorganisms is not of practical application because of energy requirements and changes in final product quality. Alternatively, chemical pasteurization is possible through mild acidification (washing first with dilute chlorine solutions, and then with acetic acid); however, this method does not prevent growth of unwanted acid-tolerand microorganisms [145]. Therefore, an interest for starter cultures able to perform a controlled fermentation by removing and/or inactivating the endogenous microbiota has arisen. The capacity of the starter culture to dominate the indigenous microbiota may be exerted via its fast growth under fermentation conditions, coupled with release of antagonistic compounds.

Several attempts to select potential starter cultures focused on their bacteriocin-production capacity have accordingly taken place; Jimenez-Díaz *et al.* [152] studied *L. plantarum* strains LPCO10 involved in Spanish-style green olive fermentation, and found two bacteriocins, viz. plantaricins S and T, with bacteriocidal activity against clostridia and propionibateria, besides being natural competitors of *L. plantarum* in olive fermentation.

Ruiz-Barba *et al.* [153] evaluated afterwards whether said strain could produce plantaricins in a natural fermentation if added as pure culture to green olive fermentation. They detected it at very low concentration by the end of fermentation, but it was probably presente throughout the whole fermentation period. Moreover, the fermentative process was similar compared with uninoculated brine, thus showing that *L. plantarum* LPCO10 may be used as a starter culture in green olive fermentation. These findings have prompted search for new bacteriocin-producer strains isolated from table olives [154-159].

In several trials encompassing food-borne bacteriocin-producer strains, it has been difficult to demonstrate bacteriocin activity – possibly because of interaction (binding) thereof with some organic compounds (*e.g.* polyphenols) in olive brines [153], or by cell repression of bacteriocin synthesis [160]. This realization implies that optimum production may require a combination of factors influencing the production of bacteriocins – so Delgado *et al.* [33] attempted to optimize bacteriocin production by *L. pentosus* B96 *in vitro* as a function of NaCl concentration and temperature, following a response surface design; these authors found that suboptimal temperature (22 °C) and moderate NaCl stress (0.65 mol l^{-1}) stimulated bacteriocin production. In a related work [161], the effect of both nutrients and medium pH upon bacteriocin ST311LD production by *Enterococcus faecium* previously isolated from spoiled black olives was assessed; optimal synthesis was detected when MRS broth was supplemented with tryptone, saccharose or vitamin C; and the optimal pH for bacteriocin production ranged in pH 5-6. Low (or no bacteriocin) activity was recorded when such strain was grown in BHI and M17 broth (or molasses).

Bacteriocin production in *L. plantarum* NC8 may apparently be activated via coculture with specific bacteria during olive fermentation [162]; expression of bacteriocin genes in many LAB is controlled via a three-component regulatory system, consisting of autoinducers — i.e. specific peptides secreted by the strain itself as extracellular signal, a histidine protein kinase and a response regulator (as part of a quorum sensing mechanism). Ruiz-Barba *et al.* [163] suggested that the presence of bacteriocin producing-inducing strains (cocultures) was the result of an environmental stimulus to switch from a constitutive to a specific adaptative response; this probably involved bacteriocin production that allowed enhanced growth and survival, and eventual ecological domination of the process.

6. Probiotic Lactic Acid Bacteria in Table Olives

The skin of olive fruit contains microscopic pores, called stomata, that are though to be the primary portals for entrance and exit of solutes and gases [164]. Their location at the interface between internal plant tissues and the environment make them convenient gates for endophytic bacteria colonization [165]; in this regard, lactic acid bacteria have been shown to enter through stomata – and predominate in the intercellular space of the sub-stomal cells [142].

The above findings disclose the spatial distribution of lactic bacteria on the fruit surface and its association in olive fermentation – thus highlighting the potential of table olives to serve as biological vectors for selected strains. Lavermicocca *et al.* [166] accordingly assessed the ability of human-borne probiotic strains, belonging to *Lactobacillus rhamnosus* (three strains), *L. paracasei* (two strains), *Bifidobacterium bifidum* (one strain) and

Bifidobacterium longum (one strain) to incorporate in, and survive on the olive surface. After a 3-month experiment, most strains showed an inconspicuous compatibility with olives, likely because they are not naturally involved in spontaneous fermentation and hardly adapted to the prevailing environmental conditions. For instance, bifidobacteria and *L. rhamnosus* GG showed a moderate survival rate until 30 days (*ca.* 10^6 CFU g^{-1}), but the population remained unchanged afterwards for *L. rhamnosus* GG – while bifidobacteria declined by *ca.* 1 log cycle; conversely, *L. paracasei* IMPC2.1 showed the highest viability (over 10^7 CFU g^{-1}) throughout the whole experiment. These data indicate suitability of table olives as vehicle to incorporate probiotics.

In order to validate table olives as bacterial conveyor matrix into the human gastrointestinal tract (GIT), five human volunteers were fed for 10 days with 10 to 15 olives per day, carrying about 10^9-10^{10} viable cells of *L. paracasei* IMPC2.1; the strain was recovered from fecal samples from four of those volunteers. The microstructure of the olive fruit surface apparently guarantees cell integrity during transit through the gastrointestinal tract [166, 167] – and international patents covering these aspects have meanwhile been issued [168]. Additionally, this strain has been tested as starter in a pilot fermentation of debittered green olives *cv.* Bella di Cerignola [140]; its persistence and efficacy were ascertained by monitoring the dynamics of the microbial population associated with the olive surface in industrial fermentation sets at 4 or 8% NaCl, and at room temperature or 4 °C.

Despite the dual role of starter and probiotic of *L. paracasei* IMPC2.1 for development of a new table olive-based probiotic product [136], most strains proposed for 'probiotication' of vegetables are from dairy origin – thus exhibiting a poor adaptation to the harsh conditions prevailing in the brine of fermented table olives [169]. Therefore, research of table olive as wild source of lactic bacteria with probiotic and technological features constitutes an emerging (and promising) field of work [2]. Previous screening for such probiotic properties as antibiotic resistance, acid and bile salt tolerance, inhibition of pathogenic bacteria, and haemolytic activity have been performed on strains that had been isolated in advance from fermented olives [117, 170]. In addition, *L. plantarum* strains isolated from Bella de Cerignola table olives have confirmed the possibility of multifunctional starters with probiotic features – including their ability to adhere to mammalian jejune epithelial cells IPEC-J2, coupled with desired technological properties [169].

Conclusion and Future Perspectives

The vast majority of the public, including medical doctors, have an incipient knowledge on the nutritional and health value of table olives – which are being replaced by unhealthier snacks, even in Mediterranean countries. Despite the high salt content of table olives, their caloric input is about half those of trivial appetizers. Furthermore, olives may supply relevant quantities of several vitamins, minerals, antioxidants and essential fatty acids. They have also high contents of beneficial fibres, and may serve as carriers of human probiotic bacteria. Claims of prophylactic, and even therapeutic actions of table olives are available, including anti-*Helicobacter pilory* and anti-colon cancer activity. Therefore, an impetus exists for expansion of the olive-based food portfolio, and to backup advertising campaigns with a stronger impact on the market of table olives.

It should be stressed that most such aspects apply only to fermented olives; the Californian process of oxidized black olives causes wash away and decay of most vitamins and antioxidants, besides being exempt of beneficial bacteria or metabolites thereof. Hence, fermented olives are still a vast and unexplored resource of potentially useful microbial strains and nutraceutical components that deserves being the object of well-structured long-term research and development programs.

ACKNOWLEDGMENTS

Project NEW PROTECTION (ref. PTDC/AGRALI/117658/2010) and doctoral fellowship (ref. SFRH/BD/81997/2011), both supervised by author F.X.M. and cosuspervised by author C.P., and funded by Fundação para a Ciência e a Tecnologia (Portugal).

REFERENCES

[1] Hasler, C. M. (2002). Functional foods: benefits, concerns and challenges – a position paper from the American Council on Science and Health. *Journal of Nutrition*, 132, 3772–3781.

[2] Peres, C., Peres, C, Hernández-Mendoza, A. and Malcata, F. X. (2012). Review on fermented plant materials, as carriers and sources of potentially probiotic lactic acid bacteria – with an emphasis on table olives. *Trends in Food Science and Technology*, 26, 31–42.

[3] Newell-McGloughlin, M. (2008). Nutritionally improved agricultural crops. *Planta Physiology*, 147, 939–953.

[4] Lombardo, N. (1988). Cultivation of the olive: a typical tree of the Mediterranean basin. *Outlook on Agriculture,* 17, 183–185.

[5] Boskou, D. (1996). *History and characteristics of the olive tree.* In *Olive Oil Chemistry and Technology*; Boskou, D., Ed.; American Oil Chemists´ Society Press: Champaign, IL, USA.

[6] IOOC (International Olive Oil Council). Statistic of Table Olive´s World Production. (2011). Assessed at: http://www.internationaloliveoil.org/ estaticos/view/132-world-table-olive-figures on 12 July 2012.

[7] Fernández-Díez, M. J., Ramos, R., Fernandez, A., Cancho, F., Pellisó, F., Vega, M., Moreno, A., Mosquera, I., Navarro, L., Quintana, M., Roldán, F., Garcia, P., and Gómez-Millán, A., (1985). *Biotecnologia de la Aceituna de Mesa.* Instituto de la Grasa y sus Derivados. Seville. Spain.

[8] Oliveira, M., Brito, D., Catulo, L., Leitão, F., Gomes, L., Silva, S., Vilas-Boas, L., Peito, A., Fernandes, I., Gordo, F. and Peres, C. (2004). Biotechnology of olive fermentation of *Galega* Portuguese variety. *Grasas y Aceites*, 55, 219–226.

[9] Covas, M. I. (2008). Bioactive effects of olive oil phenolic compounds in humans: reduction of heart disease factors and oxidative damage. *Inflammopharmacology*, 16, 216–218.

[10] IOOC (International Olive Oil Council). Statistic of Table Olive´s World Production. (2008). Assessed at: http://www.internationaloliveoil.org/ downloads/production3_ang. PDF on 12 July 2012.
[11] MADRP (2007) – Ministério da Agricultura do Desenvolvimento Rural e das Pescas. Gabinete de Planeamento e Políticas. *Anuário Vegetal 2006.*
[12] Fernández-Díez, M. J. (1983). *Biotechnology: Olives*; vol. 5, Rehm, H. J. and Reed, J. (Eds); Verlag Chemie: Weinheim, Germany; pp. 379–397.
[13] Bianchi, G. (2003). Lipids and phenols in table olives. *European Journal of Lipid Science and Technology*, 105, 229–242.
[14]] Romero, C., Brenes, M., Xousfi, K., Garcia, P., Garcia, A. and Garrido-Fernández, A. (2004). Effect of cultivar and processing method on the contents of polyphenols in table olives. *Journal of Agricultural and Food Chemistry*, 52, 479–484.
[15] Ross, R. P., Morgan, S. and Hill, C. (2002). Preservation and fermentation: past, present and future. *International Journal of Food Microbiology*, 79, 3–16.
[16] Garrido-Fernández, A., Fernández Diez, M. J. and Adams, M. R. (1997). *Table Olives: Physical and Chemical Characteristics of the Olive Fruit*. Garrido Fernández, A. *et al.* (Eds.) London, United Kingdom; Chapman and Hall; pp. 67–109.
[17] Sánchez-Gómez, A.-H., García-García, P. and Rejano, L. (2006). Elaboration of table olives. *Grasas y Aceites*, 57, 86–94.
[18] Romero, C., Garcia, P., Brenes, M., García, A., Garrido, A., (2002). Phenolic compounds in natural black Spanish olive varieties. *European Food Research Technology,* 215, 489–496.
[19] Leal-Sánchez, M. V., Ruiz-Barba, J. L., Sánchez, A. H., Rejano, L., Jiménez-Díaz, R. and Garrido, A. (2003). Fermentation profile and optimization of green olive fermentation using *Lactobacillus plantarum* LPCO10 as a starter culture. *Food Microbiology*, 20, 421–430.
[20] Steinkrauss, K. H. (1994). Nutritional significance of fermented foods. *Food Research International*, 27, 259–267.
[21] Prajapati, J. B. and Nair, B. M. (2003). The history of fermented foods, In Farnworth, E. R. (Ed.), *Handbook of Fermented Functional Foods*. CRC Press, New York; pp. 2–23.
[22] Hansen, E. B. (2002). Commerical bacterial starter cultures for fermented foods of the future. *International Journal of Food Microbiology*, 78, 119–131.
[23] Hurtado, A., Reguant, C., Esteve-Zarzoso, B., Bordons, A., and Rozès, N. (2008). Microbial population dynamics during the processing of *Arbequina* table olives. *Food Research International* 4, 738–744.
[24] Silva, T., Reto, M., Sol, M., Peito, A., Peres, C. M., Peres, C. and Malcata, F. X. (2011). Characterization of yeasts from Portuguese brined olives, with a focus on their potentially probiotic behavior. *Lebensmittel-Wissenschaft und-Technologie*, 44, 1349–1354.
[25] Damiani, P., Gobbetti, M., Cossignani, L., Simonetti, M. S. and Rossi, J. (1996). The sourdough microflora characterization of hetero- and homofermentative lactic acid bacteria, yeasts and their interactions on the basis of the volatile compounds produced. *Lebensmittel-Wissenschaft und -Technologie*, 29, 63–70.
[26] Gómez, A. H. S., García, P. G. and Navarro, L. R. (2006). Trends in table olive production. *Grasas y Aceites*, 57, 1–9.

[27] Tsapatsaris, S. and Kotzekidou, P. (2004). Application of central composite design and response surface methodology to the fermentation of olive juice by *Lactobacillus plantarum* and *Debaryomyces hansenii*. *International Journal of Food Microbiology*, 95, 157–168.

[28] Ruíz-Barba, J. L. and Jiménez-Diaz, R. (1995). Availability of essential B-group vitamins to *Lactobacillus plantarum* in green olive fermentation brines. *Applied and Environmental Microbiology*, 61, 1294–1297.

[29] Marquina, D., Peres, C., Caldas F. V., Marques, J. F., Peinado, J. M. and Spencer-Martins, I. (1992). Characterization of the yeast population in olive brines. *Letters in Applied Microbiology*, 14, 279–283.

[30] Rozès, N. and Peres, C. (1996). Effect of oleuropein and sodium chloride on viability and metabolism of *Lactobacillus plantarum*. *Applied Microbiology and Biotechnology*, 45, 839–843.

[31] Rozès, N. & Peres, C. (1998). Effects of phenolic compounds on the fatty acid composition of *Lactobacillus plantarum. Applied Microbiology and Biotechnology*, 49, 108-111.

[32] Maldonado, A., Ruíz-Barba, J. L., Belén-Floriano, Jiménez-Díaz, R. (2002). The locus responsible for production of plantaricin S, a class IIb bacteriocin produced by *Lactobacillus plantarum* LPCO10, is widely distributed among wild-type *L. plantarum* strains isolated from olive fermentations. *International Journal of Food Microbiology*. 77, 117–124.

[33] Delgado, A., Brito, D., Peres, C., Noé-Arroyo, F. and Garrido-Fernández, A. (2005). Bacteriocin production by *Lactobacilllus pentosus* B96 can be expressed as a function of temperature and NaCl concentration. *Food Microbiology*, 22, 521–528.

[34] Delgado, A., Noé-Arroyo, F., Brito, D., Peres, C., Fevereiro, P. and Garrido-Fernández A. (2007). Optimum bacteriocin production by *Lactobacillus plantarum* 17.2b requires absence of NaCl and apparently follows mixed metabolite kinetics. *Journal of Biotechnology*, 130, 193–201.

[35] WHO (2009). Advisory Group on Integrated Surveillance of Antimicrobial Resistance (AGISAR). *Critically Important Antimicrobials for Human Medicine (2nd revision)*. Geneva, World Health Organization, (http://www.who.int/foodsafety/foodborne_disease/ CIA_2nd_rev_2009.pdf, accessed 9 April 2012).

[36] de Keersmaecker, S. C. J., Verhoeven, T. L. A., Desair, J., Marchal, K., Vanderleyden, J. and Nagy, I. (2006). Strong antimicrobial activity of *Lactobacillus rhamnosus* GG against *Salmonella typhimurium* is due to accumulation of lactic acid. *FEMS Microbiology Letters*, 259, 89–96.

[37] Gotteland, M., Brunser, O. and Cruchet, S. (2005). Systematic review: are probiotics useful in controlling gastric colonization by *Helicobacter pylori*? *Alimentary Pharmacology*, 23, 1077–1086.

[38] Myllyluoma, E. (2007). *The role of probiotics in* Helicobacter pylori *infection*. PhD thesis. Institute of Biomedicine and Pharmacology. University of Helsinki, Finland.

[39] Lopes, A. I., Oleastro, M., Palha, A., Fernandes, A. and Monteiro, L. (2005). Antibiotic-resistant *Helicobacter pylori* strains in Portuguese children. *Pediatric Infectious Disease Journal*, 24, 404–409.

[40] Garrido-Fernández, A. and Lopez-Lopez, A., (2008). Revalorización nutricional de la Aceituna de Mesa. Oral communication. *II Jornadas Internacionales de la Aceituna de Mesa.* Seville. 26-27 March 2008.

[41] Cunha, S., Ferreira, I. M. P. L. V. O., Fernandes, J. O., Faria, M. A., Beatriz, M. and Oliveira, P. P. (2001). Determination of lactic, acetic, succinic and citric acids in table olive by HPLC/UV. *Journal of Liquid Chromatography and Related Technologies*, 24, 1029–1038.

[42] Viola, P. and Viola, M. (2009). Virgin olive oil as a fundamental nutritional component and skin protector. *Clinical Dermatology,* 27, 159–165.

[43] Guerfel, M., Ben-Mansour, M., Ouni, Y., Guido, F., Boujnah, D. and Zarrouk, M. (2012). Triacylglycerols composition and volatile compounds of virgin olive oil from Chemlali cultivar: comparison among different planting densities. *The Scientific World Journal.* 2012, 1–6.

[44] Salas, J. J., Sanchéz, J., Ramli, U. S., Manaf, A. M., Willians, M. and Harwood, J. L. (2000). Biochemistry of lipid metabolism in olive and other oil fruits. *Progress in Lipid Research*, 39, 151–180.

[45] López-López, A., Montaño, A., Ruíz-Méndez, M. V. and Garrido-Fernández, A. (2008). Sterols, fatty alcohols, and triterpenic alcohols in commercial table olives. *Journal of the American Oil Chemists' Society*, 85, 253–262.

[46] López-López, A., Rodríguez Gómez, F. Cortés-Delgado, A. and Garrido-Fernández, A. (2009). Changes in sterols, fatty alcohol and triterpenic alcohol during ripe olive processing. *Czech Journal of Food Science*, 27, S225–S226.

[47] Lavelli, V. and Bondesan, L. (2005). Secoiridoids, tocopherols, and antioxidant activity of monovarietal extra virgin olive oils extracted from destoned fruits. *Journal of Agricultural and Food Chemistry*, 53, 1102–1107.

[48] Guillén, R., Heredia, A., Felizoón, B., Jiménez, A., Montaño, A., and Fernández-Bolanños, J. (1992). Fibre fraction carbohydrates in *Olea europeae* (*Gordal* and *Manzanilla* var.). *Food Chemistry*, 44, 173–174.

[49] Sanz, C., Luaces, P., and Perez, A. G. (2007). Processing of olive fruit for enhancement of carotenoid level in virgin olive oil. *Acta Horticulturae*, 744, 377–380.

[50] Arroyo-López, F. N., Querol, A., Bautista-Gallego, J. and Garrido-Fernández, A. (2008). Role of yeasts in table olive production. *International Journal of Food Microbiology*, 10, 189–196.

[51] Abbas, C. A. (2006). Production of antioxidants, aromas, colours, flavours, and vitamins by yeasts. In *Yeasts in Food and Beverages*. Querol, A. and Fleet, H., Eds. Springer–Verlag, Berlin, pp. 285–334.

[52] López-López, A., García, P. and Garrido-Fernandez, A. (2008). Multivariate characterization of table olives according to their mineral nutrient composition. *Food Chemistry*, 106, 369–378.

[53] Naczk, M. and Shahidib, F. (2004). Extraction and analysis of phenolics in food. *Journal of Chromatography A*, 1054, 95–111.

[54] Covas, M. I., Nyyssonen, K. and Poulsen, H. E. (2006). The effect of polyphenols in olive oil on heart disease risk factors. *Annals of Internal Medicine*, 145, 333–431.

[55] Boskou, D., Blekas, G., and Tsimidou, M. (2005). Phenolic compounds in olive oil and olives. *Current Topics in Nutraceutical Research*, 3, 125–136.

[56] Baldioli, M., Servili, M., Perretti, G. and Montedoro, G. F. (1996). Antioxidant activity of tocopherols and phenolic compounds of virgin olive oil. *Journal of the American Oil Chemists' Society*, 73, 1583–1593.

[57] Cody, V., Middleton, E., Harborne, J. B. and Beretz, A. (1988). Biology and medicine: plant flavonoids. II – Biochemical, cellular and medicinal properties. In *Progress in Clinical and Biological Research*, vol. 280, Alan R. Liss, New York.

[58] Blekas, G., Vassilakis, C., Harizanis, C., Tsimidou, M. and Boskou, D. G. (2002). Biophenols in table olives. *Journal of Agricultural and Food Chemistry*, 50, 3688–3692.

[59] Montedoro, G. F. (1972). Phenolic constituents of virgin olive oils. Identification of some phenolic acids and their antioxidant capacity. *Scienze degli Technologie Alimentari*, 3, 177–186.

[60] Soler-Rivas, C., Espín, J. C. and Wichers, H. J. (2000). Oleuropein and related compounds. *Journal of the Science of Food and Agriculture*, 80, 1013–1023.

[61] Amiot, M. J., Fleuriet, A. and Macheix, J. J. (1986). Importance and evolution of phenolic compounds in olive during growth and maturation. *Journal of Agricultural and Food Chemistry*, 34, 823–826.

[62] Tripoli, E., Giammanco, M., Tabacchi, G., di Majo, D., Giammanco, S. and La Guardia, M. (2005). The phenolic compounds of olive oil: structure, biological activity and beneficial effects on human health. *Nutrition Research Reviews*, 18, 98–112.

[63] Pereira, J. A., Pereira, A. P. G., Ferreira, I. C. F. R., Valentão, P., Andrade, P. B., Seabra, R., Estevinho, L. and Bento, A. (2006). Table olives from Portugal: phenolic compounds, antioxidant potential, and antimicrobial activity. *Journal of Agricultural and Food Chemistry*, 54, 8425–8431.

[64] Rovellini, P., Cortesi, N. and Fedeli, E. (1997). Analysis of flavonoids from *Olea europaea* by HPLC-UV and HPLC-electrospray-MS. *Rivista Italiana delle Sostanze Grasse*, 74, 273–279.

[65] Brenes, M., García, A., Rios, J. J., García, P. and Garrido-Fernández, A. (2002). Use of 1-acetoxypinoresinol to authenticate *Picual* olive oils. *International Journal of Food Science and Technology*, 37, 615–625.

[66] Visioli, F. and Galli, C. (2002). Biological properties of olive oil phytochemicals. *Critical Reviews in Food Science and Nutrition*, 42, 209–221.

[67] Matalas, A.-L., Zampelas, A., Stavrinos, V., and Wolinsky, I. (2001). *The Mediterranean Diet: Constituents and Health Promotion*; CRC Press: Boca Raton, FL, USA.

[68] Frankel, E. N. (2011). Nutritional and biological properties of extra virgin olive oil. *Journal of Agricultural and Food Chemistry*, 59, 785–792.

[69] Covas, M. I., Nyyssonen, K., Poulsen, H. E., Kaikkonen, J., Zunft, H. J., Kiesewetter, H., Gaddi, A., de la Torre, R., Mursu, J., Baumler, H., Nascetti, S., Salonen, J. T., Fito, M., Virtanen, J. and Marrugat, J. (2006). EUROLIVE Study Group. The effect of polyphenols in olive oil on heart disease risk factors: a randomized trial. *Annals of Internal Medicine*, 145, 333–341.

[70] Hashim, Y. Z., Eng, M., Gill, C., McGlynn, H. and Rowland, I. R. (2005). Components of olive oil and chemoprevention of colorectal cancer. *Nutrition Reviews*, 63, 374–86.

[71] Escrich, E., Solanas, M., Moral, R. and Escrich R. (2011). Modulatory effects and molecular mechanisms of olive oil and other dietary lipids in breast cancer. *Current Pharmaceutical Design*, 17, 813–830.

[72] Delgado-Lista, J., Garcia-Rio, A., Perez-Martinez, P., Lopez-Miranda, J. and Perez-Jimenez, F. (2011). Olive oil and haemostasis: platelet function, thrombogenesis and fibrinolysis. *Current Pharmaceutical Desing*, 17, 778–785.

[73] Lucas, L., Russell, A. and Keast, R. (2011). Molecular mechanisms of inflammation. Anti-inflammatory benefits of virgin olive oil and the phenolic compound oleocanthal. *Current Pharmaceutical Design*, 17, 754–768.

[74] Teissedre, P. L., Frankel, E. N., Waterhouse, A. L., Peleg, H., and German, J. B. (1996). Inhibition of *in vitro* human LDL oxidation by phenolic antioxidants from grapes and wines. *Journal of the Science of Food and Agriculture*, 70, 55–61.

[75] Battinelli, L., Daniele, C., Cristiani, M., Bisignano, G., Saija, A. and Mazzanti, G. (2006). *In vitro* antifungal and anti-elastase activity of some aliphatic aldehydes from *Oleae europaea* L. fruit. *Phytomedicine*, 13, 558–563.

[76] Romero, C., Medina, E., Vargas, J., Brenes, M. and Castro, A. D. (2007). *In vitro* activity of olive oil polyphenols against *Helicobacter pylori. Journal of Agricultural and Food Chemistry*, 55, 680–686.

[77] Furneri, P. M., Marino, A., Saija, A., Uccella, N. and Bisignano, G. (2012). *In vitro* antimycoplasmal activity of oleuropein. *International Journal of Antimicrobial Agents*, 20, 293–296.

[78] Tuck, K. L. and Hayball, P. J. (2002). Major phenolic compounds in olive oil: metabolism and health effects. *Journal of Nutritional Biochemistry*, 13, 636–644.

[79] Mascitelli, L., Pezzetta, F. and Goldstein, M. R. (2010). Is the beneficial antioxidant effect of olive oil mediated by interaction of its phenolic constituents and iron? *Archives on Medical Research*, 41, 295–296.

[80] de Lucas, C. R. (2011). What is the nutritional value of green olives? (2011). Assessed at: http://www.livestrong.com/article/241576-what-is-the-nutritional-value-of-green-olives/ #ixzz219f22joh on 26 July 2012.

[81] Biala, D. (2011). What vitamins and minerals do olives have? Assessed at: http://www.livestrong.com/article/370210-what-vitamins-minerals-do-oliveshave/ #ixzz219iJjWiW on 2 October 2012.

[82] Jiménez, A., Rodrı́guez, R., Fernández-Caro, I., Guillén, R., Fernández-Bolaños, J. and Heredia, A. (2000). Dietary fibre content of table olives processed under different European styles: study of physico-chemical characteristics. *Journal of the Science of Food and Agriculture*, 80, 1903–1908.

[83] Rodríguez, R., Jiménez, A., Fernández-Bolaños, J., Guillén, R., and Heredia, A. (2006). Dietary fibre from vegetable products as source of functional ingredients. *Trends in Food Science and Technology*, 17, 3–15.

[84] Conde, C., Delrot, S. and Geros, H. (2008). Physiological, biochemical and molecular changes occurring during olive development and ripening. *Journal of Plant Physiology*, 165, 1545–1562.

[85] Hernández, A., Martín, A., Córdoba, M. G., Benito, M. J., Aranda, E. and Pérez-Nevado, F. (2007). Identification and characterization of yeast isolated from the elaboration of seasoned green table olives. *Food Microbiology*, 24, 346–351.

[86] López, A., Montaño, A., García, P. and Garrido-Fernández, A. (2006). Fatty acid profile of table olives and its multivariate characterization using unsupervised (PCA) and supervised (DA) chemometrics. *Journal of Agricultural and Food Chemistry*, 54, 6747–6753.

[87] Grundy, S. M. (1986). Comparison of monounsaturated fatty acids and carbohydrates for lowering plasma cholesterol. *New England Journal of Medicine*, 314, 745–748.

[88] Ranalli, A. and Angerosa, F. (1996). Integral centrifuges for olive oil extraction. The qualitative characteristics of products. *Journal of American Oil Chemists' Society*, 73, 417–422.

[89] Han, S. N., Adolfsson, O., Lee, C. K., Prolla, T. A., Ordovas, J., and Meydani, S. N. (2006). Age and vitamin E-induced changes in gene expression profiles of T cells. *Journal of Immunology*, 177, 6052–6061.

[90] Kochhar, S. P. (2001). *Frying improving quality: the composition of frying oils*. Rossel, J.B., Ed: Woodhead Publishing: Cambridge, UK; pp. 87–114.

[91] Miles, E. A., Zoubouli, P. and Calder, P. C. (2005). Differential anti-inflammatory effects of phenolic compounds from extra virgin olive oil identified in human whole blood cultures. *Nutrition*, 21, 389–394.

[92] Prades, J., Vögler, O., Alemany, R., Gomez-Florit, M., Funari, S. S., Ruiz-Gutiérrez, V. and Barceló, F. (2011). Plant pentacyclic triterpenic acids as modulators of lipid membrane physical properties. *Biochimica et Biophisica Acta*, 1808, 752–760.

[93] Romero, C., García, A., Medina, E., Ruíz-Méndez, M. V., de Castro, A. and Brenes, M. (2010). Triterpenic acids in table olives. *Food Chemistry*, 118, 670–674.

[94] Juan, M. E., Wenzel, U., Ruiz-Gutierrez, V., Daniel, H. and Planas, J. M. (2006). Olive fruit extracts inhibit proliferation and induce apoptosis in HT-29 human colon cancer cells. *Journal of Nutrition*, 136, 2553–2557.

[95] Juan, M. E., Planas, J. M., Ruiz-Gutierrez, V., Daniel, H. and Wenzel, U. (2008). Antiproliferative and apoptosis-inducing effects of maslinic and oleanolic acids, two pentacyclic triterpenes from olives, on HT-29 colon cancer cells. *British Journal of Nutrition*, 100, 36–43.

[96] Xu, H. X., Zeng, F. Q., Wan, M. and Sim, K. Y. (1996). Anti-HIV triterpene acids from *Geum japonicum*. *Journal of Natural Products*, 59, 643–645.

[97] Moneriz, C., Marín-García, P., García-Granado, A., Bautista, J. M., Diez, A. and Puyet, A. (2011). Parasitostatic effect of maslinic acid. I. Growth arrest of *Plasmodium falciparum* intraerythrocytic stages. *Malaria Journal*, 10, 10–82.

[98] Kris-Etherton, P. M., Hecker, K. D., Bonanome, A., Coval, S. M., Binkoski, A. E. Hilpert, K. F., Griel, A. E., and Etherton, T. D. (2002). Bioactive compounds in foods: their role in the prevention of cardiovascular disease and cancer. *American Journal of Medicine*, 113, 71S–88S.

[99] Visioli, F., Galli, C., Plasmati, E., Viappiani, S., Hernandez, A., Colombo, C. and Sala, A. (2000). Olive phenol hydroxytyrosol prevents passive smoking-induced oxidative stress. *Circulation*, 102, 2169–2171.

[100] Ghabbour, N. Lamzira, Z., Thonart, P., Peres, C., Markaoui, M. and Asehraou, A. (2011). Selection of oleuropein-degrading lactic acid bacteria strains isolated from fermenting Moroccan green olives. *Grasas y Aceites*, 62, 84–89.

[101] Jenner, P. and Olanow, C. W. (1996). Oxidative stress and the pathogenesis of Parkinson's disease. *Neurology*, 47, 161S–170S.

[102] Ryan, D. and Robards, K. (1998). Phenolic compounds in olives. *Analyst*, 123, 31R–44R.

[103] Ho, P. W. L., Ho, J. W. M., Hui-Fang, L., So, D. H. F., Tse, Zero, H. M. Chan, K.-H., Ramsden, D. B. and Ho, S.-L. (2012). Mitochondrial neuronal uncoupling proteins: a target for potential disease-modification in Parkinson's disease. *Translational Neurodegeneration*, 1, 3–50.

[104] Pitt, J., Roth, W., Lacor, P., Blankenship, M., Velasco, P., de Felice, F., Breslin, P. A. and Klein, W. L. (2009). Alzheimer's-associated A-β oligomers show altered structure, immunoreactivity and synaptotoxicity with low doses of oleocanthal. *Toxicology and Applied Pharmacology*, 240, 189–197.

[105] González-Correa, J. A., Navas, M. D., Lopez-Villodres, J. A., Trujillo, M., Espartero, J. L. and de la Cruz, J. P. (2008). Neuroprotective effect of hydroxytyrosol and hydroxytyrosol acetate in rat brain slices subjected to hypoxia-reoxygenation. *Neuroscience Letters*, 446, 143–146.

[106] Manna, C., Migliardi, V., Golino, P., Scognmiglio, A., Galetti, P., Chiariello, M. and Zappia, V. (2004). Oleuropein prevents oxidative myocardial injury by ischemia and reperfusion. *Journal of Nutrition and Biochemistry*, 15, 461–468.

[107] Benkhalti, F., Prost, J., Paz, E., Perez-Jimenez, F., el Modafar, C. and el Boustani, E. (2002). Effects of feeding virgin olive oil or their polyphenols on lipid of rat liver. *Nutrition Research*, 22, 1067–1075.

[108] Auroma, O. I., Deiane, M., Jenner, A., Halliwell, B., Kaur, M., Banni, S., Corongiu, F. P., Dess, M. A. and Aesbach, R. (1998). Effects of hydroxytyrosol found in extra virgin olive oil on oxidative DNA damage and on low-density lipoprotein oxidation. *Journal of Agricultural and Food Chemistry*, 46, 5181–5187.

[109] Papadopoulos, G. and Boskou, D. (1991). Antioxidant effect of natural phenols on olive oil. *Journal of the American Oil Chemists' Society*, 68, 669–671.

[110] Zrelli, H., Matsuoka, M., Kitazaki, S., Araki, M., Kusunoki, M., Zarrouk, M. and Miyazaki, H. (2011). Hydroxytyrosol induces proliferation and cytoprotection against oxidative injury in vascular endothelial cells: role of Nrf2 activation and HO-1 induction. *Journal of Agricultural and Food Chemistry*, 59, 4473–4482.

[111] Saleh, N. K. and Saleh, H. A. (2011). Olive oil effectively mitigates ovariectomy-induced osteoporosis in rats. *BMC Complementary and Alternative Medicine*, 11, 10–20.

[112] Tassou, C. C. and Nychas, G. J. E. (1994). Inhibition of *Staphylococcus aureus* by olive phenolics in broth and in a model food system. *Journal of Food Protection*, 57, 120–124.

[113] Tassou, C. C. and Nychas, G. J. E. (1995). Inhibition of *Salmonella enteritidis* by oleuropein in broth and in a model food system. *Letters in Applied Microbiology*, 20, 120–124.

[114] Capasso, R., Evidente, A., Schivo, L., Orru, G., Marcialis, M. A. and Cristinzio, G. (1995). Antibacterial polyphenols from olive oil mill waste waters. *Journal of Applied Bacteriology*, 79, 393–398.

[115] Hirschman, S. Z. (1972). Inactivation of DNA polymerases of murine leukaemia viruses by calcium elenolate. *Nature: New Biology*, 238, 277–279.

[116] Gourama, H. and Bullerman, L. B. (1987). Effects of oleuropein on growth and aflatoxin production by *Aspergillus parasiticus*. *Lebensmittel-Wissenschaft und - Technologie*, 20, 226–228.

[117] Owen, R. W., Giacosa, A., Hull, W. E., Haubner, R., Spiegelhalder, B. and Bartsch, H. (2000). The antioxidant/anticancer potential of phenolic compounds isolated from olive oil. *European Journal of Cancer*, 36, 1235–1247.

[118] Olive Oil Times (2012). Assessed at http://www.oliveoiltimes.com/olive-oil-health-benefits on 15 July 2012.

[119] Salvini, S., Sera, F., Caruso, D., Giovannelli, L., Visioli, F., Saieva, C., Masala, G., Ceroti, M., Giovacchini, V., Pitozzi, V., Galli, C., Romani, A., Mulinacci, N., Bortolomeazzi, R., Dolara, P. and Palli, D. (2006). Daily consumption of a high-phenol extra-virgin olive oil reduces oxidative DNA damage in postmenopausal women. *British Journal of Nutrition*, 95, 742–51.

[120] Sánchez-Villegas, A., Verberne, L., de Irala, J., Ruíz-Canela, M., Toledo, E., Serra-Majen, L., and Martínez-González, M. A. (2011). Dietary fat intake and the risk of depression: the SUN project. *PLoS ONE* 6, 8–22.

[121] Kellie, L., Tuck, P. and Hayball, J. (2002). Major phenolic compounds in olive oil: metabolism and health effects. *The Journal of Nutritional Biochemistry*, 13, 636–644.

[122] Visioli, F., Galli, C., Bornet, F., Mattei, A., Patelli, R., Galli, G. and Caruso, D. (2000). Olive oil phenolics are dose-dependently absorbed in humans. *FEBS Letters*, 468, 159–160.

[123] Covas, M. I. (2007). Olive oil and the cardiovascular system – Review. *Pharmaceutical Research*, 55, 175–186.

[124] Ghanbari, R., Anwar, F., Khalid, M., Alkharfy, Anwarul-Hassan, G. and Saari, N. (2012). Valuable nutrients and functional bioactives in different parts of olive (*Olea europaea* L.) – a review. *International Journal of Molecular Science*, 13, 3291–3340.

[125] Lima, J. T., Almeida, J. R., Barbosa-Filho, J. M., Assis, T. S., Silva, M. S., da-Cunha E. V. L., Braz-Filho, R. and Silva, B. A. (2005). Spasmolytic action of diplotropin, a furanoflavan from *Diplotropis ferruginea* Benth., involves calcium blockade in ginea-pig ileum. *Zeitschrift für Naturforschung* – B, 60, 1093–1100.

[126] di Carlo, G., Autore, G., Izzo, A. A., Maiolino, P., Mascolo, N., Viola, P., Diurno, M. V. and Capasso, F. (1993). Inhibition of intestinal motility and secretion by flavonoids in mice and rats: structure-activity relationships. *Journal of Pharmacy and Pharmacology*, 45, 1054–1059.

[127] Sumbul, S., Mohd, A. A., Mohd, A. and Mohd, A. (2011). Role of phenolic compounds in peptic ulcer: an overview. *Journal of Pharmacy and Bioallied Science*, 3, 361–367.

[128] di Carlo, G., Mascolo, N., Izzo, A. A. and Capasso, F. (1999). Flavonoids: old and new aspects of a class of natural therapeutic drugs. *Life Sciences*, 64, 337–53.

[129] Dekanski, D., Janicijevic-Hudomal, S., Tadic, V., Markovic, G., Arsic, I. and Dusan, M. M. (2009). Phytochemical analysis and gastroprotective activity of an olive leaf extract. *Journal of Serbian Chemical Society*, 74, 367–77.

[130] de la Puerta, R., Ruíz-Gutiérrez, V. and Hoult, J. R. (1999). Inhibition of leukocyte 5-lipoxygenase by phenolics from virgin olive oil. *Biochemical Pharmacology*, 57, 445–449.

[131] Lee-Huang, S., Lin-Huang, P., Zhang, D., Lee, J. W., Bao, J., Sun, Y., Chang, Y. T., Zhang, J. and Huang, P. L. (2007). Discovery of small-molecule HIV-1 fusion and integrase inhibitors oleuropein and hydroxytyrosol: Part I. Fusion [corrected] inhibition. *Biochemical and Biophysical Research Communications*, 354, 872–878.

[132] Hsu, C. L. and Yen, G. C. (2008). Phenolic compounds: evidence for inhibitory effects against obesity and their underlying molecular signaling mechanisms. *Molecular Nutrition and Food Research*, 52, 53–61.

[133] Novelli, E. L. B., Santos, P., Assalin, H., Souza, G., Rocha, K., Ebaid, G., Seiva, F., Mani, F. and Fernandes, A. (2009). N-acetylcysteine in high sucrose induced obesity: energy expenditure, metabolic shifting for cardiac health. *Pharmacology Research*, 59, 74–79.

[134] Daeschel, M. A. and Fleming, H. P. (1984). Selection of lactic acid bacteria for use in vegetable fermentations. *Food Microbiology*, 1, 303–313.

[135] Corsetti, A., Perpetuini, G., Schirone, M., Tofalo, R. and Suzzi, G. (2012). Application of starter cultures to table olive fermentation: an overview on the experimental studies. *Frontiers in Microbiology*, 3, 1-6.

[136] Sisto, A. and Lavermicocca, P. (2012). Suitability of a probiotic *Lactobacillus paracasei* strain as a starter culture in olive fermentation and development of the innovative patented product "probiotic table olives". *Frontiers in Microbiology*, 3, 1–5.

[137] Botta, C. and Cocolin, L. (2012). Microbial dynamics and biodiversity in table olive fermentation: culture-dependent and -independent approaches. *Frontiers in Microbiology*, 3, 1–10.

[138] Randazzo, C. L., Restuccia, C., Romano, A. D. and Caggia, C. (2004). *Lactobacillus casei*, dominant species in naturally fermented Sicilian green olives. *International Journal of Food Microbiology*, 90, 9–14.

[139] Ercolini, D., Villani, F., Aponte, M. and Mauriello, G. (2006). Fluorescence *in situ* hybridisation detection of *Lactobacillus plantarum* group on olives to be used in natural fermentations. *International Journal of Food Microbiology*, 112, 291–296.

[140] de Bellis, P., Valerio, F., Sisto, A., Lonigro, S. L. and Lavermicocca, P. (2010). Probiotic table olives: Microbial populations adhering on olive surface in fermentation sets inoculated with the probiotic strain *Lactobacillus paracasei* IMPC2.1 in an industrial plant. *International Journal of Food Microbiology*, 140, 6–13.

[141] Hurtado, A., Reguant, C., Bordons, A. and Rozès, N. (2012). Lactic acid bacteria from fermented table olives. *Food Microbiology*, 31, 1–8.

[142] Nychas, G.-J. E., Panagou, E. Z., Parker., M. L., Waldron, K. W. and Tassou, C. C. (2002). Microbial colonization of naturally black olives during fermentation and associated biochemical activities in the cover brine. *Letters in Applied Microbiology*, 34, 173–177.

[143] Medina, E., Gori, C., Servili, M., de Castro, A., Romero, C. and Brenes, M. (2010). Main variables affecting the lactic acid fermentation of olives. *International Journal of Food Science and Technology*, 45, 1291–1296.

[144] Brenes, M. (2004). Olive fermentation and processing: Scientific and technological challenges. *Journal of Food Science*, 69, 33–34.

[145] Lanza, B., Zago, M., Carminati, D., Rossetti, L., Meucci, A., Marfisi, P., Russi, F., Iannucci, E. and di Serio, M. G. (2012). Isolation and preliminary characterization of *Lactobacillus plantarum* bacteriophages from table olive fermentation. *Annals of Microbiology*, 62, 419–426.

[146] Marsilio, V., Saghetti, L., Lannucci, E., Russi, F., Lanza, B. and Felicioni, M. (2005). Use of a lactic acid bacteria starter culture during green olive (*Olea europaea* L. cv *Ascolana tenera*) processing, *Journal of the Science of Food and Agriculture*, 85, 1084–1090.

[147] Servili, M., Settanni, L., Veneziani, G., Esposto, S., Massitti, O., Taticchi, A., Urbani, S., Montedoro, G. F. and Corsetti, A. (2006). The use of *Lactobacillus pentosus* 1MO to shorten the debittering process time of black table olives (cv. *Itrana* and *Leccino*): a pilot-scale application. *Journal of Agricultural and Food Chemistry*, 54, 3869–3875.

[148] Aponte, M., Blaiotta, G., Croce, F. L., Mazzaglia, A., Farina V, Settanni, L. and Moschetti, G. (2012). Use of selected autochthonous lactic acid bacteria for Spanish-style table olive fermentation. *Food Microbiology*, 30, 8–16.

[149] Kumral, A., Basoglu, F. and Sahin, I. (2009). Effect of the use of different lactic starters on the microbiological and physicochemical characteristics of naturally black table olives of *Gemlik* cultivar. *Journal of Food Processing and Preservation*, 33, 651–664.

[150] Sánchez, A.-H., Rejano, L., Montaño, A. and de Castro, A. (2001). Utilization at high pH of starter cultures of lactobacilli for Spanish-style green olive fermentation. *International Journal of Food Microbiology*, 67, 115–122.

[151] Ciafardini, G., Marsilio, V., Lanza, B. and Pozzi, N. (1994). Hydrolysis of oleuropein by *Lactobacillus plantarum* strains associated with olive fermentation. *Applied and Environmental Microbiology*, 60, 4142–4147.

[152] Jiménez-Díaz, R., Rios-Sánchez, R. M., Desmazeaud, M., Ruíz-Barba, J. L. and Piard, J.-C. (1993). Plantaricins S and T, two new bacteriocins produced by *Lactobacillus plantarum* LPCO10 isolated from a green olive fermentation. *Applied and Environmental Microbiology*, 59, 1416–1424.

[153] Ruíz-Barba, J. L., Cathcart, D. P., Warner, P. J. and Jiménez-Díaz, R. (1994). Use of *Lactobacillus plantarum* LPCO10, a bacteriocin producer, as a starter culture in Spanish-style green olive fermentations. *Applied and Environmental Microbiology*, 60, 2059–2064.

[154] Lavermicocca, P., Gobbetti, M., Corstti, A. and Capulo, L. (1998). Characterization of lactic acid bacteria isolated from olive phylloplane and table olive brines. *Italian Journal of Food Science*, 10, 27–39.

[155] Delgado, A., Brito, D., Fevereiro, P., Peres, C. and Marques-Figueiredo, J. (2001). Antimicrobial activity of *L. plantarum*, isolated from a traditional lactic acid fermentation of table olives. *Le Lait*, 81, 203–215.

[156] Kacem, M., Zadi-Karam, H. and Karam, N.-E. (2005). Detection and activity of plantaricin OL15, a bacteriocin produced by *Lactobacillus plantarum* OL15 isolated from Algerian fermented olives. *Grasas y Aceites*, 56, 192–197.

[157] Kacem, M., Zadi-Karam, H. and Karam, N.-E. (2006). Testing of *Lactobacillus plantarum* isolates isolated from fermented green olives for their inhibitory activity against lactic acid bacteria and characterization of a bacteriocin-like substance produced by *L. plantarum* OT2 isolate. *Dirasat: Pure Sciences*, 33, 224–234.

[158] Fazeli, M. R., Vaghari, E., Jamalifar, H., Ebrahim, Z. and Samadi, N. (2009). Antimicrobial activity of *Lactobacillus plantarum* strains isolated from fermented olives origin. *Journal of Medicinal Plants*, 8, 14–18.

[159] Shafighi, M., Emami, Z., Shahsanaei, M. and Khaliliyan, E. (2012). Antibacterial activity of lactic acid bacteria isolated from table olives against skin pathogens. *World Academy of Science, Engineering and Technology,* 61, 930–933.

[160] Nilsen, T., Nes, I. F. and Holo, H. (1998). An exported inducer peptide regulates bacteriocin production in *Enterococcus faecium* CTC492. *Journal of Bacteriology,* 180, 1848–1854.

[161] Todorov, S. D. and Dicks, L .M. T. (2005). Optimization of bacteriocin ST11LD production by *Enterococcus faecium* ST311LD, isolated from spoiled black olives. *The Journal of Microbiology*, 43, 370–374.

[162] Maldonado, A., Jiménez-Díaz, R. and Ruíz-Barba, J. L. (2004). Induction of plantaricin production in *Lactobacillus plantarum* NC8 after coculture with specific Gram-positive bacteria is mediated by an autoinduction mechanism. *Journal of Bacteriology,* 186, 1556–1564.

[163] Ruíz-Barba, J. L., Caballero-Guerrero, B., Maldonado-Barragán, A. and Jiménez-Díaz, R. (2010). Coculture with specific bacteria enhances survival of *Lactobacillus plantarum* NC8, an autoinducer-regulated bacteriocin producer, in olive fermentations. *Food Microbiology*, 27, 413–417.

[164] Proietti, P., Famiani, F. and Tombesi, A. (1999). Gas exchange in olive fruit. *Photosynthetica*, 36, 423–432.

[165] Gudesblat, G. E., Torres, P. S. and Vojnov, A. A. (2009). Stomata and pathogens warfare the gates. *Plant Signalin and Behavior*, 4, 1114–1116.

[166] Lavermicocca, P., Valerio, F., Lonigro, S. L., De Angelis, M., Morelli, L., Callegari, M.L., Rizzello, C. G. and Visconti, A. (2005). Study of adhesion and survival of lactobacilli and bifidobacteria on table olives with the aim of formulating a new probiotic food. *Applied and Environmental Microbiology,* 71, 4233–4240.

[167] Lavermicocca, P. (2006). Highlights on new food research. *Digestive and Liver Disease*, 38, S29–S299.

[168] Lavermicocca, P., Lonigro, S. L., Visconti, A., de Angelis, M., Valerio, F. and Morelli, L. (2007). Table olives containing probiotic microorganisms. *International Patent* WO2005053430 (A1); US2007086990 (A1); EP1843664 (A0); CA2546776 (A1).

[169] Bevilacqua, A., Altieri, C., Corbo, M. R., Sinigaglia, M. and Ouoba, L. I. I. (2010). Characterization of lactic acid bacteria isolated from Italian *Bella di Cerignola* table olives: selection of potential multifunctional starter cultures. *Journal of Food Science*, 75, M536–M544.

[170] Chiu, H.-H., Tsai, C.-C., Hsih, H.-Y. and Tsen, H.-Y. (2008). Screening in pickled vegetables for potential probiotic strains of lactic acid bacteria able to inhibit the *Salmonella* invasion in mice. *Journal of Applied Microbiology*, 104, 605–612.

In: Functional Foods
Editors: Aron Robinson and Dominick Emerson
ISBN: 978-1-62417-435-3

Chapter 3

MEDITERRANEAN DIET: FUNCTIONAL FOODS AND PHYSICAL ACTIVITY, BENEFITS FOR HUMAN HEALTH

Anita Ferraretto*[*], *Silvia Perego and Amelia Fiorilli
Dipartimento di Scienze Biomediche per la Salute, Università degli Studi di Milano, Italy

ABSTRACT

The Mediterranean diet is a well recognized life and food habits having relevant association with a reduced mortality caused by diseases such as cardiovascular disease, obesity, diabetes, cancer and neurodegenerative disorders. The importance of a healthy balanced diet lies on the fact that benefits come from the presence and the interaction of almost all the nutrients with which it is composed. It is a matter of fact that single nutrients can behave differently from what it is observed when they are all mixed together with interactive possibility. Under this perspective, the Mediterranean diet is both composed by a great number of single functional food and, as a whole, it is a result of a balance between the single nutrient properties, as evidenced by its great capacity to prevent all the chronic degenerative disorders above mentioned. Among the functional food present in the Mediterranean diet are cereals, legumes, fruit and vegetables, nuts, olive oil as the prevalent fats for dressing, red wine in moderate quantity and consumed at meals, fish and poultry as the main source of protein and polyunsaturated/saturated fats, modest quantity of dairy products, spices. Since the Mediterranean diet is a dietary pattern common to more than one country in the Mediterranean basin, some differences can be found between the food consumed by the populations. The health benefits coming from the food of the Mediterranean diet resides on the presence of bioactive compounds such as polyphenols, carotenoids, phytosterols, fibers, monounsaturated and polyunsaturated fatty acids, displaying antioxidant activity, protection from cancer and hypertension, improvement of the immune response. Due to the presence of more than one functional food groups in the same dietary pattern, sometimes in the same meal, diverse species of polyphenols as well as of phytosterols, fibers and fatty acids can be combined and activated. Next to the positive properties derived from the food, the

[*] Corresponding author: Dipartimento di Scienze Biomediche per la Salute, LITA, via Fratelli Cervi 93, Segrate (Milano), Università degli Studi di Milano, anita.ferraretto@unimi.it.

physical activity also account for an important aspect of this life habits. In fact, since lifestyle modification programs provide a method to change eating and activity habits, any diet intervention becomes more valid with a regular daily physical activity.

The last element characterizing the Mediterranean diet is the perception of a meal as a moment to spend with other people and of food as a positive link. For all these complex and heterogeneous aspects, the Mediterranean diet has recently been named as "intangible cultural heritage by UNESCO".

INTRODUCTION

It is a matter of fact that food and life habits can influence both positively and negatively our health. This assumption is the result of a lot of studies during the last decades having as a subject the composition of a whole diet, as the Mediterranean Diet (MD), or some specific component, as the amount of fats and/or protein, in relation to the most widespread pathologies. The results of these studies underlined as, besides the energy balance and the nutrients of the diet, the benefits coming from one type of diet rather than others is due to the presence of some food components possessing additional roles to that of being micro or macronutrients, for instance the antioxidant activity of vitamin C and E, thus affecting our body health. Under this perspective, diet becomes a tool to get or maintain the body fitness. Food, either natural or formulated, displaying these abilities were named "functional food", while the chemicals, naturally present in food and responsible of the beneficial effects on health, are named "nutraceuticals". While the pharmacological industries are interested to the nutraceuticals for their use in the alternative medicine, the food industry is deeply interested to develop a market of functional foods so that new and old products can be sold with the appealing to act in that way.

In the present chapter the nutraceuticals and the functional foods known to be present and to characterize the MD are been reviewed with a special attention to the composition of the Italian MD. The concept of MD has been developed by the observation arisen in the Seven Country Studies [1] in which the food habits have been correlated with the death incidence for coronary heart diseases in the population of the Mediterranean countries compared to the population of North Europe. From this point of view, MD cannot be considered as a precise list of foods to be consumed rather than a lifestyle, in which the dietary pattern coexists with a moderate physical activity and meals preparation and consumption are realized with pleasure. The dietary recommendation which characterizes the Italian MD are schematically presented in Figure 1, while the functional foods and nutraceuticals contained are reported in Figure 2.

PART I: NUTRACEUTICALS

Phenolic Compounds

These molecules represent an heterogeneous class of micronutrients abundant in vegetables of which they represent secondary metabolites secreted by the same plants toward aggression caused by pathogens or ultraviolet radiations. They are responsible of the browning and the changed quality, in particular organoleptic characteristics, of vegetable food due to their oxidation. From the structural point of view polyphenols can be classified according to the number of phenol rings they contain, but also on the basis of the association between these rings and the carbohydrates and organic acids, or the association between them. All the phenols can be originated from the benzoic acid or the cinnamic acid. Derivates of the benzoic acid are tannins and simple phenols, such as those present in tea (gallic acid) and in some red fruits, black radish and onion, but overall they are not common in food. Conversely, the cinnamic acid derivatives are more common in food in which they can be present in a glycosylated form [2]. Molecules such as flavonoids, stilbenes and lignans belong to this group. Flavonoids are the most studied and known compounds, they include flavonols (quercetin, kaempferol..), flavones (glycosides of luteolin and apigenin), flavanones, isoflavones (genistein, daidzein, glycitein), flavanols (catechins, proanthocyanidins), anthocyanins. Among the stilbenes, resveratrol represents the most extensively studied molecule, its effects at cellular level are wide, as a consequence its role as antioxidant seems to be involved in the prevention of cardiovascular diseases and the progression of degenerative disorders. Moreover, recent studies has clarified a new equally important role of resveratrol on glucose homeostasis and obesity [3]. Lignans are found in the linseed which represent the main source together with cereals, vegetables (garlic, asparagus, carrots) and fruits (pears, prunes).

Fruits, vegetables, tea, coffee and red wine represent common sources of polyphenols, but their variable content and above all the different degree of bioavailability from polyphenol to polyphenol are the cause of the different activity exerted in our body and of the difficulty to recognize a precise target of action. In general, polyphenols once coniugated with glycine, glucuronic acid and sulfate are hydrolyzed by the gut microbiota and absorbed by the intestine in the form of aglycones. The most recent studies recognized a role for polyphenols as potent antioxidants thus they are involved in the modulation of different enzymes and cell activities linked to diseases such as cancer, cardiovascular and neurodegenerative pathologies [4, 5].

Isoprenoids

Isoprenoids are a group of plant metabolites displaying various functions, from the participation in the plant cellular processes to the physiologically activities, such as photosynthesis and seed germination [6]. Carotenoids, saponins, tocotrienols, tocopherols and simple terpenes belong to this group, all characterized by a high degree of heterogeneity in their chemical structure. The presence of these molecules in the human diet is warranted by the consume of vegetables and fruits and the effects on human health are still a matter of discussion, even if some mechanism has been elucidated.

Carotenoids, notably β-carotene, lycopene, zeaxanthin and lutein, besides showing pro vitamin A activity (β-carotene), are known as antioxidants, though their bioavailability, depending by the food matrix and the co-ingested food characteristics as well as by the host characters [7], could condition the real benefits for humans. As potent antioxidants they are involved in reducing DNA damage, malignant transformation, and all other processes linked to certain types of cancer and degenerative diseases, such as ischemic heart disease and cataract. Their importance in the process of aging is also well known, as well as their ability to enhance immunity and increase intercellular communication [8]. Specifically, β-carotene and lycopene from a tomato-rich diet exert a protection for skin, while zeaxanthin and lutein exert a protection for the macula. A role in the modulation of redox signaling, leading to gene expression, was recently recognized to lycopene [9].

Tocopherols and tocotrienols constitute two isoforms of vitamin E, the tocopherols are saturated forms whereas the tocotrienols are unsaturated forms. Tocopherols are present in the most plant leaves and seeds, tocotrienols are present in only a very small fraction of plants, both isoforms of vitamin E are been detected in human milk. They act as antioxidants, particularly tocopherols regulate reactive-oxygen species, cell signaling and oxidative damage. Recent studies have indicated that tocotrienols exhibit also antiproliferative, antisurvival, proapoptotic, antiangiogenic, and anti-inflammatory activities, with health outcomes as anticancer, cardioprotective, and neuroprotective effects [10-12].

Saponins are another group of plant natural products having a function in the pathogen resistance. They consisted of triterpene or steroid aglycone bound to one or more sugar chains. Their application in the cosmetics and pharmacological field is wide. The most known saponins are the ones extracted by the ginger root. Ginseng saponins or ginsenosides are the main active principals of ginseng. To ginseng was attributed an anticancer potentiality due to the presence of ginsenosides, in fact recent clinical and preclinical studies have indicated these compounds as new agents in the treatment of primary and metastatic tumors [13].

Carbohydrates

Carbohydrates can be separated into two basic groups based upon their digestibility in the gastrointestinal (GI) tract. The group of starch, simple sugars, and fructans is easily hydrolyzed by enzymatic reactions and absorbed in the small intestine. These compounds can be referred to as non-structural carbohydrates or simple carbohydrates. The group of cellulose, hemicellulose, lignin, pectin and β-glucans is resistant to digestion in the small intestine though it undergoes bacterial fermentation in the large intestine. These compounds can be referred to as complex carbohydrates or non-starch polysaccharides.

Among the latter, β-glucan is the predominant non-starch polysaccahride of cell walls in cereal grains such as barley and oats. It is composed of glucose molecules with mixed β-(1→4) and β-(1→3) bonds. This specific chemical structure is responsible for physical properties, such as viscosity and solubility, as well as the potential to influence cholesterol metabolism [14].

A large number of studies indicated the effectiveness of β-glucan against various diseases and disorders and several reported applications underline its tendency to reduce onset of colorectal cancer, to increase stool bulk and provide assistance against constipation, to reduce glycemic index, to reduce serum cholesterol levels, to produce short-chain fatty acids and promote the growth of beneficial gut microflora [15-19].

Concerned with the source, barley β-glucan was more effective in the regulation of glucose and insulin responses compared to oat β-glucan, while oat β-glucan may reduce total blood and low-density lipoprotein (LDL) cholesterol levels [19]. In fact, it was noticed that β-glucan containing extrudates from oat displays the ability to bind and replenish the deficiency of bile acids, as a consequence more cholesterol from the body is consumed for the synthesis of bile acids thus lowering the serum cholesterol level in the body. Furthermore, oat β-glucan may increase fecal excretion of bile acids and enhance hepatic conversion of cholesterol into bile acids [20].

Consumption of a diet high in barley β-glucan has been shown to prevent insulin resistance and can be used for diabetic patients; in fact, the β-glucan containing diet promotes hepatic insulin signaling by decreasing serine phosphorylation of insulin receptor [21].

Pectin is a linear polymer of galacturonic acid connected with α (1→4) bonds. It is a water soluble polysaccharide that bypasses enzymatic digestion of the small intestine but is easily degraded by the microflora of the colon.

Inside the GI pectin maintains the ability to form a gel or thicken a solution. This is thought to be the likely mechanism behind its many beneficial effects on health including improved cholesterol and lipid metabolism [22]. Several recent clinical studies demonstrated that oral pectin supplementation to children and infants reduced acute intestinal infections and significantly slowed diarrhea [23]. The mechanism of action seems to be a reduction in pathogenic bacteria such as *Shigella, Salmonella* and *Enterobacter*, as supported by Olano-Martin et al. [24] who observed that pectin stimulates the growth of certain strains of *Bifidobacteria* and *Lactobacillus in vitro.*

Bran is the outer most layer of a cereal grain that have been shown to display an effect on postprandial glucose levels, serum cholesterol, colon cancer, and body mass, although the efficacy of bran may change due to its source. Qureshi et al. [25] found that subjects suffering type I and II diabetes decreased their fasting glucose levels due to the daily consumption of 10 g of stabilized rice bran over two months. The results may be due to an increased intestinal viscosity, but is more likely a result of a decreased carbohydrate/caloric intake. In addition to a possible effect on carbohydrate absorption and metabolism, bran also seems to have the same effect on lipids; in fact in the same study Qureshi et al. [25] found that 10 g of rice bran consumed for eight weeks was able to decrease serum total cholesterol, LDL cholesterol and triglycerides. The reduction in cholesterol level is likely due to an increase in bile acid synthesis.

Resistant starches (RS) are defined as any starch not digested in the small intestine. RS behave like soluble fiber without sacrificing palatability and mouth feel, thus resistant starch tries combining the health benefits of dietary fiber/whole grain with the sensory feel of refined carbohydrates. A majority of human studies involving RS have shown a decrease in postprandial blood glucose and insulin levels. Behall et al. [26] found that women consuming a range between 0.7-5 g of RS had significantly lower postprandial glucose and insulin levels when compared to the control. However, this study failed to maintain an equal amount of available carbohydrate between the treatments and control. Several studies report that longer term consumption of a RS may decrease fasting cholesterol and triglyceride levels; an effect supposed to be due to the increased intestinal viscosity [27].

Proteins

High-quality protein sources are meat, fish, eggs and dairy products, good sources are beans and peas, while moderately good sources are the grains, namely rice, wheat and corn.

Dietary guidelines at the international level recommend diets with a high energy intake from carbohydrates, a low energy intake from fat and an even lower energy intake from protein. However, there has long been interest in the ideal balance of these energy sources to achieve better health, including the ideal proportion of proteins in the diet [28]. Santesso et al. compared higher- and lower-protein diets by reviewing many randomized controlled trials [29]. The authors found evidence (of a moderate quality) that higher-protein diets had no significant effects or no effect at all on surrogate cardiovascular disease outcome, namely blood pressure, total cholesterol, LDL cholesterol and C-reactive protein (CRP). However, what they did observe was a small positive effect on HDL cholesterol and a moderate triglyceride reduction with higher-protein diets, although the effect was smaller when the lower risk of bias studies were separately analyzed. The results corroborate studies suggesting that higher-protein diets may result in better lipid profiles, although the effects are likely to be small [30]. The results of the meta-regression also suggest that the lower carbohydrate content of the higher-protein diet contributes to this positive change, though the marked differences in the protein intake were not positively associated with better HDL profiles. There was some evidence to suggest an effect of higher-protein diets on outcomes related to diabetes: glycosylated haemoglobin (HbA_{1c}) and fasting blood glucose.

There have been reports on a relation between major dietary protein source and incident coronary heart disease in women [31]. Indeed, a higher intake of red meat and whole-fat dairy products has been associated with a higher risk of coronary heart disease, whereas a higher intake of nuts, fish and poultry were associated with a lower risk [32]. The comparison was made with the same number of servings per day. Changing round protein sources in the diet may contribute to stroke prevention.

Low carbohydrate-high protein diets could have a short term effect on weight control [33, 34]. However concern has been expressed with respect to cardiovascular outcomes. Although low carbohydrate-high protein diets may be nutritionally acceptable if the protein is mainly of plant origin, and reduced carbohydrates limits the carbohydrates to simple and refined ones, these guidelines are not always recognized and acted upon by the general public [35].

Lipids and Fatty Acids

The primary essential fatty acid is linoleic acid (LA, 18:2n-6), which forms the basis of the n-6 family. LA owes its predominance to the fact that it is the most common PUFA in the dynamic phospholipids (especially lecithin) needed for membrane structure and for the lipoproteins involved in lipid transport, particularly HDL. LA can be elongated and desaturated to form 20 carbon fatty acids, such as arachidonic acid (AA, 20:4n-6). These fatty acids act together on structural lipids and cell signals and are responsible for the control of the many cell activities found in daily life. In fact, epidemiological evidence supports a dietary role of LA in reducing the risk of coronary heart disease (CHD). Indeed, a cross-population study (all healthy men) from four European populations [36] found that high LA adipose tissue, a marker of dietary LA intake, was associated with lower CHD mortality. Furthermore, it has been found that serum LA is negatively related to cardiovascular mortality in post-infarction middle-aged men [37], while a low dietary LA intake predisposed the subjects to myocardial infarction [38]. Hegsted and Ausman [39] studied dietary factors impacting CHD in men from 18 countries (with PUFA intake ranging from 1.4% to 11%), and found that dietary PUFA was negatively associated with CHD mortality after adjusting for saturated fatty acid (SFA) intake. LA is the most potent dietary fatty acid for reducing plasma total cholesterol (TC) and LDL cholesterol, both CHD risk factors. It has been clearly demonstrated in human that diets extremely high in LA, i.e. providing 16% to 29% LA, significantly lowered LDL cholesterol plasma by 16-22%, compared to diets high in saturated fatty acids (19% to 30% SFA) and low in LA (only 2.3%-4.5%). With regard to LA action mechanisms, it has been noted that LA-rich fats enhance LDL hepatic receptor-dependent clearance and concomitantly reduce LDL cholesterol production.

Alpha-linolenic acid (LNA, 18:3n-3) is the second primary essential fatty acid that can be elongated and desaturated to form highly specialized 22-carbon fatty acids within the n-3 family. It has been suggested that dietary LNA (and its subsequent metabolic end products) could protect against CHD [40, 41]. Control studies revealed an association between high adipose tissue LNA content and a lower risk of myocardial infarction. Indeed, dietary LNA intake was significantly associated with lower CHD mortality and mortality from other causes. Studies on male and female populations revealed that LNA provides some protection against cardiac deaths and non fatal myocardial infarction, regardless of other factors [42]. There is increasing evidence that diets with modest amounts of eicosapentaenoic acid (EPA, 20:5 n-3) and docosahexaenoic acid (DHA, 22:6 n-3), LNA conversion products found in oily fish, decrease the risk of ischemic heart disease. Furthermore, high serum and adipose tissue n-3 longer-chain polyunsaturated fatty acid have been associated with a reduced risk of acute or fatal myocardial infarction (MI). The consumption of one or more servings of fish per week has been associated with a 52% lower risk of sudden cardiac death, compared to less than one fish meal /month. Both EPA and DHA are potent hypotriacylglycerolemic agents, and administering 3 g/d of EPA + DHA to normolipemic subjects, or patients with elevated triglycerides (TGs), reduces plasma TGs by 12% and 21% respectively, compared to placebo administration.

Thus the balance of n-6 and n-3 fatty acids in the diet has a critical influence on cardiovascular health. Indeed, it has been suggested that an intake of about 6% for LA, 0.75% for LNA, and 0.25%-0.5% for EPA+DHA would be adequate for most healthy adults. This corresponds to an n-6:n-3 ratio of about 6:1.

n-6 PUFA derived eicosanoids have pro-inflammatory and immunoactive functions, whereas n-3 PUFA derived eicosanoids have anti-inflammatory properties, traditionally attributed to their ability to inhibit the formation of n-6 PUFA-derived eicosanoids. It has been shown that increasing the n-3 to n-6 fatty acid ratio in the diet favors EPA production in the body, or increasing the dietary EPA and DHA intake through the consumption of fatty fish or fish-oil supplements reduces the incidence of many chronic diseases that involve inflammatory processes, namely cardiovascular diseases, inflammatory bowel disease, cancer and rheumatoid arthritis, but also psychiatric and neurodegenerative illness [43].

Prebiotics

Prebiotics are defined as "selectively fermented ingredients that allow specific changes, both in the composition and/or activity of the gastrointestinal microbiota that confer benefits upon host well-being and health" [44]. According to this definition to be classified as prebiotic a food ingredient has to i) resist gastric acidity, hydrolysis by mammalian enzymes and gastrointestinal absorption; ii) be fermented by the intestinal microbiota and iii) selectively stimulate the growth and/or activity of intestinal bacteria associated with health and wellbeing.

Established prebiotics include fructans, galacto-oligosaccharides and lactulose [44]. Additionally, a number of oligosaccharides have been identified, which may qualify as prebiotics once sufficient evidence is established. Fructans, which are chains of fructofuranose residues linked by β2 > 1 linkages, include plant-extracted inulin, as well as lower molecular weight fructo-oligosaccharides (FOS). Galacto-oligosaccharides (GOS) are complex oligosaccharides produced from lactose by galactosyl transfer reactions. The synthetic sugar lactulose is produced by alkaline isomerization of lactose. Additionally, particular types of β-glucans have recently been shown to exert prebiotic effects, especially by enhancing the growth of *Lactobacilli* in the gastrointestinal tract [45].

Many of these established prebiotic compounds are part of a common diet. Fructans are found in many vegetables including e.g. leek, onion and artichoke, while commercially available inulin (used as food and feed ingredient) is produced from chicory root, which is very rich in this polymer. GOS are naturally occurring in human milk.

Several studies in infants and children consistently show a decrease in the incidence of common childhood diarrhea after dietary supplementation with FOS, GOS or a mixture of both [46-48]. Other studies show no effect on diarrheal incidence, but report a reduction in the duration and/or severity of the infections [49]. In addition to the effects exerted through modulation of the gut microbiota, prebiotics may protect against pathogens through direct interactions with them. Several studies with different types of preparations of GOS consistently show that this prebiotic has the potential in vitro to reduce adherence of enteropathogenic *E. coli*, as well as *Salmonella* to epithelial cell lines [50, 51]. Additionally, GOS was shown to provide protection against murine infection with *Salmonella* when administrated immediately prior to challenge, which indicates that the protective effect was a result of blocking of pathogen adhesion rather than of modification of the microbiota [50].

Several dietary fibers, including several fibers possessing prebiotic properties, have been shown to hold immune modulating activities, both in *in vitro* and *in vivo* studies. Indirect effects of prebiotics on the immune system may be caused by stimulation of the growth of probiotic bacteria or by stimulation of the production of short chain fatty acids (SCFA). The increase in the production of SCFA by the gut microbiota upon ingestion of prebiotics is well established [52] and the SCFA produced in the intestinal tract may affect both the epithelial cells and the immune system cells.

Studies on the effects of prebiotics on host microbiota should not focus only on selected bacterial groups considered to be beneficial, such as *Bifidobacteria* and *Lactobacilli*, but should increasingly take into account the effects on the microbiota as a whole. Moreover, research on the health benefits of prebiotics is likely to expand to health benefits beyond microbiota modulation. Already, the efficacy of prebiotics is being investigated in areas such as allergy prevention and mineral absorption. Reduction of the risk of infections and protection against pathogens are additionally among the future targets of prebiotic research.

Probiotics

Probiotics are defined "viable microorganisms, sufficient amounts of which reach the intestine in an active state and thus exert positive health effects" [53]. Probiotic microorganisms do not act exclusively in the large intestine via affecting the intestinal flora. They also affect other organs, either by modulating immunological parameters, intestinal permeability and bacterial translocation, or by providing bioactive or otherwise regulatory metabolites.

The majority of probiotic microorganisms belong to the genera *Lactobacillus* and *Bifidobacterium*. However, other bacteria and some yeasts may have probiotic properties as well (*Enterococcus, Streptococcus thermophilus, Saccharomyces boulardii*). *Lactobacilli* and *Bifidobacteria* are Gram positive lactic acid-producing bacteria that constitute a major part of the normal intestinal microflora in animals and humans [54].

Lactobacilli are non-spore forming rod-shaped bacteria. They have complex nutritional requirements and are strictly fermentative, aerotolerant or anaerobic, aciduric or acidophilic. They are found in a variety of habitats where rich, carbohydrate-containing substrates are available, such as human and animal mucosal membranes, on plants or material of plant origin, sewage and fermented milk products fermenting or spoiling food.

Bifidobacteria constitute a major part of the normal intestinal microflora in humans throughout life. They appear in the stools a few days after birth and increase in number thereafter. They are non-motile, non-sporulating rods with varying appearance. Most strains are strictly anaerobic.

The yeast *Saccharomyces boulardii*, used in pharmaceutical products, was shown to exert beneficial effects against diarrhea, and *Enterococcus* containing pharmaceuticals are used in pediatrics.

Most health effects attributed to probiotic microorganisms are related, directly or indirectly, i.e. mediated by the immune system, to the gastrointestinal tract. The mechanisms and the efficacy of a probiotic effect often depend on interactions with the specific microflora of the host or immunocompetent cells of the intestinal mucosa.

Many strains of probiotic bacteria have been shown i) to modulate (temporarily) the intestinal microflora and/or ii) to inhibit colonization of the gut by (potential) pathogens, as well as iii) translocation of pathogenic bacteria through the intestinal wall and the infection of other organs. Suggested, but unconfirmed mechanisms for these effects include: reduced intestinal pH, production of bactericidal substances (e.g. organic acids, H_2O_2), agglutination of pathogenic microorganisms, strengthening barrier function of the intestinal mucosa, competition for fermentable substrates or receptors on the cellular surface of the mucosa, release of gut-protective (arginine, glutamine, short chain fatty acids, conjugated linoleic acid (CLA) and absorption and metabolization of potentially pathogenic, toxic, or cancerogenic metabolites and enzymes, modulation of immunologic mechanisms, or stimulation of the intestinal motility and mucus production [54].

Well-established probiotic effects are: prevention and/or reduction of duration and complaints of rotavirus-induced or antibiotic-associated diarrhea as well as alleviation of complaints due to lactose intolerance [55-57].

Reduction of the concentration of cancer-promoting enzymes and/or putrefactive (bacterial) metabolites in the gut [58-60]. Prevention and alleviation of unspecific and irregular complaints of the gastrointestinal tracts in healthy people; beneficial effects on microbial aberrancies, inflammation and other complaints in connection with: inflammatory diseases of the gastrointestinal tract, Helicobacter pylori infection or bacterial overgrowth [61-63]. Prevention or alleviation of allergies and atopic diseases in infants [64, 65]. Prevention of respiratory tract infections (common cold, influenza) and other infectious diseases as well as treatment of urogenital infections [66, 67].

All the nutraceuticals associated to the MD are reported in Figure 2.

Part II: Food

Fruits and Vegetables

This food group which constitutes the base of the Italian MD (Figure 1) represents the main source of polyphenols, one of the reason to consume more than 2 portion of fruits and vegetables daily. Due to the different types of phenols contained and to their multiplicity of action at body level the suggestion is to vary the choice of this food every day, a simple but very important recommendation to benefit of all and different properties. Black and blueberries, strawberry, kiwi, cherry, apricot, apple, pear an all the other types of fruits are considered as sources of antioxidants due to their high content of polyphenols. A special consideration is to be made about soy. Soy isoflavones are characterized by a high bioavailability and the property to bind to estrogen (ER)-β receptors, thus affecting cell signaling.

The known outcomes of soy consumption for human health are a reduction in the hot flushes and in bone resorption in menopausal women [5], together with the antioxidant properties. Green vegetables also contain a considerable amount of lutein, β-carotene, and β-cryptoxanthin: carrots and pumpkins are the best sources of α-carotene; red bell peppers, oranges, potatoes, broccoli, and green vegetables together with carrots are the main sources of β-carotene. β-cryptoxanthin is present at low concentration, its main sources are tropical fruits like papaya. Tomato, watermelon and pink grapefruit are the main sources of lycopene. Green vegetables such as spinach, Brussels sprouts, broccoli and peas contain lutein, while zeaxanthin is found in high concentrations in egg yolks and corn.

Wine

Though wine, especially red wine, cannot be considered as a needful nutrient, its daily consume, if in moderate quantity (see the Italian MD pyramid, Figure 1) and during the main meals, can be considered positive due to content of polyphenols, expecially resveratrol. The specific reported benefits from a moderate consume of red wine are: a positive profile in the lipoproteins, in coagulation and platelet aggregation, in oxidative mechanisms and in endothelial functions [68], with a vasorelaxatory effect involving a nitric oxide pathway. Since its discovery in 1997, resveratrol, which is present in berries and lignified plant tissues as well as in grapes, was considered as a promising therapeutic tool for a lot of pathologies. This consideration arose from the observation that population used to consume moderate quantity of red wine together with a high fat diet was characterized by a diminished incidence of cardiovascular diseases with respect to population consuming the same diet but devoid of red wine, a phenomenon known as “French paradox”. At present the explanation of this phenomenon is based on the complex dietary features and life habits of those population, besides the only consume of red wine.

Interesting and new potentialities have been described for resveratrol in the control of glucose homeostasis, type 2 diabetes, obesity and aging [69, 70], even if the doses used in the in vitro experimentation sometimes seem not attainable with a human diet, a consideration which deserves more investigations.

Spices

Spices are common condiments in the MD, and their daily use is usually recommended by dietitians and experts in nutrition in order to avoid salt but confer a good taste to food. There are no doubts that all the phenol compounds are present in the different species of spices, from the flavonoids to the caffeic acid [71]. The well known properties of spices are: antibacterial, anti-inflammatory, antioxidant, moreover they act as anti carcinogen, as inhibitors of platelet aggregation, stimulate digestion, are protective toward diabetes and hypertension. Spices can also act in reducing lipid absorption and increasing cholesterol excretion. Recent studies have also revealed a positive role for black pepper, ginger and capsaicin of chili in maintaining the energetic balance thus the body weight [72]. Spices in food favor the digestive processes, increasing the secretion of saliva and gastric juices [73], the concentration of biliary acids and increasing the secretion of digestive enzymes in the pancreas, such as lipase, amylase, trypsin, and chemotrypsin [73]. The beneficial properties vary from spice to spice and probably it could have synergic effects, with increasing health-related potential.

Cereals and Whole Cereals

Cereal grains are an important energy source throughout the world. Grain-based foods provide the majority of the carbohydrate and dietary fiber intakes in many countries. In the European Prospective Investigation into Cancer and Nutrition (EPIC) study populations, 27% of total carbohydrate intake was from bread [74]. The majority of bread, as well as other baked goods, is made of refined white wheat flour, devoid of the outer grain layers rich in cell wall material and associated phenolic compounds, minerals and vitamins. Epidemiological studies constantly show that intake of whole grain and cereal dietary fiber protects against the rapidly increasing chronic diseases related to a sedentary lifestyle, such as cardiovascular disease and type 2 diabetes [75, 76]. In fact, whole grains are inherently rich in dietary fiber, containing ~80% more dietary fiber than refined grains. Furthermore, as a consequence of the refining process, there are substantial losses in essential minerals, vitamins, and phytonutrients [77].

Whole grains are rich sources of vitamins, minerals, dietary fiber, lignans, β-glucan, inulin, numerous phytochemicals, phytosterols, phytin, and sphingolipids [77]. The bran contains phenolic compounds, vitamins, minerals, and fiber; the endosperms, the largest component of the whole grain, contains carbohydrates (starch), protein, vitamins, and minerals. Adom et al. [78] reported that the majority of the beneficial phytochemicals are present in the bran and germ fractions of whole grains. Whole grains contain fiber, RS, oligosaccharides, and lignans, which have important biological activities and functions [77]. For example, the dietary fiber, RS, and oligosaccharides in whole grains may contribute to cholesterol reduction, healthy blood glucose and insulin concentrations, improved digestive health, and lower risk of certain gastrointestinal cancers [79]. Lignans found in whole grains have strong antioxidant and phytoestrogenic effects. Intestinal microflora play a role in converting these plant lignans into the mammalian lignans, enterolactone and enterodiol, which may provide protection against chronic diseases such as hormone-related cancers, diabetes, and heart disease [77, 79].

Antinutrients such as phytic acid, tannins, and enzyme inhibitors are also present in whole grains and may contribute to their overall protective effects. Phytic acid forms chelates with various metals suppressing iron-catalyzed redox reactions and associated oxidative damage.

Cross-sectional and prospective epidemiological studies indicate that the regular consume of whole grains is associated with reduced risk of obesity and weight gain [80]. Several mechanisms have been suggested to explain why whole grain intake may play a role in body weight management. Fiber content of whole grain foods may influence food volume and energy density, gastric emptying, and glycemic response. It has also been proposed that they play an important role in promoting satiety; individuals who eat more whole grain foods may eat less because they feel satisfied with less food. The current evidence among a predominantly Caucasian population suggests that consuming 3 or more servings of whole grains per day is associated with lower BMI, lower abdominal adiposity, and with trends toward lower weight gain over time [81].

Epidemiological studies from North American and European cohorts have consistently shown that consumption of whole grains is associated with reduced risk of cancer and cardiovascular disease CVD [82]. A number of mechanisms have been suggested for the coronary heart disease risk reduction associated with whole grains. These mechanisms include: the soluble fiber component that is associated with increased fecal excretion of cholesterol and bile acid; the antioxidant and anti-inflammatory properties, possibly due to the presence of polyphenolics and other phytonutrients in whole grains; the fermentation of whole grain polysaccharides in the large bowel resulting in propionate production, which can inhibit cholesterol synthesis and the increased serum enterolactone concentrations from fermentation of plant lignans by the gut microflora [77, 79, 82]. Other potential mechanisms include the modulation of blood glucose and insulin responses, the improvement of vascular function and blood pressure, and weight control. Higher whole grain intake has been associated with reduced risk of hypertension [83]. In addition to fiber, whole grains contribute nutrients such as protein, magnesium, and potassium, which have been shown to play a role in blood pressure reduction. Many dietary components can positively affect gastrointestinal health, including fiber, RS, oligosaccharides, phytochemicals, antioxidant vitamins, and minerals. Of the myriad of foods available, whole grains provide most of these beneficial components. They play an important role in digestive health and this is attributed to not only the fiber component but also to the other nutrients and phytonutrients present. Whole grains contain a significantly higher proportion of nutrients than their refined grain counterparts.

Dietary Fiber

Dietary fiber is a carbohydrate that resists digestion and absorption and may or may not undergo microbial fermentation in the large intestine. This definition is essentially the basis to its correlation between consumption levels and possible health benefits.

Dietary fiber contain a unique blend of bioactive components including resistant starches, vitamins, minerals, phytochemicals and antioxidants. As a result, research regarding their potential health benefits has received considerable attention in the last several decades. Epidemiological and clinical studies demonstrate that consumption of dietary fiber and whole grain intake is inversely related to obesity, type II diabetes, cancer and CVD [84-86]. Recent studies support the inverse relationship between dietary fiber and the development of several types of cancers including colorectal, small intestine, oral, larynx and breast [87].

Dietary fiber and whole grains are an abundant source of nutrients including vitamins, minerals, and a slowly digestible energy. In addition, they contain phytochemicals such as phenolics, carotenoids, lignans, β-glucan and inulin; these chemicals, secreted by plants, are important factors in human health.

The synergistic effect of phytochemicals, increased nutrient content and digestive properties, are believed to be the mechanism behind dietary fibers beneficial effects on the treatment and prevention of obesity and diabetes, reduced CVD and decreased incidence of certain types of cancer [84, 88, 89]. Fibers can affect glucose metabolism by interfering with release and absorption of glucose in the small intestine. Soluble viscous fibers are especially related to attenuated absorption of glucose but insoluble cereal fiber has also been shown to improve insulin sensitivity [90].

Dietary fibers ability to decrease body weight or attenuate weight gain could be contributed to several factors: i) soluble fiber, when fermented in the large intestine, produces glucagon-like peptide (GLP-1) and peptide YY (PYY), two gut hormones which play a role in inducing satiety [91]; ii) dietary fiber may significantly decrease energy intake [84]. Women who consumed increased levels of fiber tended to also have a decreased consumption of dietary fat.

A large amount of research has reported an inverse relationship between fiber consumption and the risk for coronary heart disease and several types of cancer. The mechanisms behind these findings are still unclear. However, it is thought to be attributed to several factors including increasing bile acid excretion, decreased caloric intake, increased short chain fatty acid production, carcinogen binding effects, increased antioxidants, and increased vitamins and minerals [27]. The digestive and viscosity characteristics of dietary fiber are thought to be responsible of their effects on diabetes and obesity risk. These mechanisms appear to decrease nutrient absorption, therefore, decreasing metabolizable energy. Dietary fiber may also be able to decrease gross energy of a food due to its lower energy density.

Dairy Products

Milk and dairy products, not only cow's milk but also that of sheep, goats and buffalos are part of a healthy MD. Indeed, the fat and protein content of the milk of the various animal species differs only slightly, that is of high priority in human nutrition, the protein being of high nutritional value. Such protein is found in the casein and whey and depends on both the essential aminoacids and the metabolism of the animal. Whey protein has high lysine levels, sulfur containing aminoacids, methionine, cystein, tryptophan and threonine, which all depend on the dietary protein source. It has already been demonstrated that the protein in milk has native or latent biological functionality. Indeed, the bioactive molecules found during ripening and digestion include casomorphins, lactoferrin, casokinins, immunopeptides, casoplatelins and phosphopeptides. Thus milk is not only a source of nitrogen and essential aminoacids but it also contains bioactive peptides that are released during digestion and processing.

Table 1. Composition of various cheese types [92]

Cheese type	Protein (g/100 g)	Fat (g/100 g)	Ca (g/100 g)	P (g/100 g)	Milk source	Ripening
Parmesan	33.5	28.1	1.16	0.685	cow	Up to 2-3 years
Mozzarella	18.7	19.5	0.16	0.35	buffalo, cow	unripened
Provolone	28.1	28.2	0.72	0.52	cow	ripened
Ricotta	10.5	17.3	0.34	0.38	Whey	unripened
Feta	15.6	20.2	0.36	0.28	sheep, goat, cow	10 to 15 days
Mascarpone	7.6	47	0.68	0.97	cow	unripened
Pecorino	25.8	32	0.6	0.59	sheep, goat	ripened

Unfortunately milk is a perishable product, but humans have long been able to convert it into cheese products with a longer shelf-life but that still contain high nutrient levels. Furthermore, milk is a very good source of bioavailable calcium, as shown in Table 1.

Italian cheeses such as Parmesan, Pecorino and Grana Padano take a long time to mature, and during the ripening there is most likely the formation of bioactive peptides. Instead soft cheeses like mozzarella and provolone are called "pasta filata", being cut into small pieces, warmed and kneaded to form a continuous matrix. Their ripening period is very limited, due to non-inactivated enzymes, and they are mostly consumed unripened. They contain the casein fraction, a precursor of some bioactive peptides.

Bioactive Peptides

Opiate, antithrombotic and anti-hypertension activities, immune-modulation and mineral utilization are all activities exerted by many peptides.

Opioid peptides can be considered to be like enkephalins, this means that they have an affinity for opiate receptors and result in opiate-like effects, they act by binding to specific receptors of the target cells. Individual receptors are responsible for specific physiological effects such as emotional behavior and the suppression of intestinal motility (μ-receptors), emotional behavior (σ-receptors), sedation and food intake (κ-receptors). Whey proteins contain an opioid-like sequence.

It was shown by de Leeuw that Angiotensin converting enzyme (ACE)-inhibitory peptides have anti-hypertensive properties [93]. The authors reported that dairy peptides lowered blood pressure in a dose-dependent way in a mildly hypertensive patient. Indeed, ACE inhibition could influence different regulatory systems as the peptides are located in different tissues throughout the body.

The glycomacropeptide (GMP), which occurs during digestion, appears to limit clot formation as it inhibits von Willebrand factor dependent platelet aggregation. Indeed, it has been suggested that GMP could be given to humans intravenously or orally to prevent thrombosis [94].

The peptides coming from the casein digestion and named casein phosphopeptides (CPPs) are able to bind minerals such as calcium and iron and are known as mineral carriers.

Numerous studies both *in vitro* and *in vivo* [95] have studied the possibility to address to CPPs a specific potential in the calcium absorption process at intestinal level, with successfully results *in vitro* but with some doubts to be solved *in vivo*. Moreover, recent data described an involvement of CPPs in the modulation of the intestinal immune system by triggering cytokine secretion and stimulating IgA production, in the release of IL-6 cytokine in human epithelial intestinal cell lines, besides the modulation of cell proliferation and apoptosis in different human cell cultures [96].

Hydrophobic peptides derived from milk protein can inhibit bacterial growth. They are present in casein and whey proteins and show antimicrobial activity. Instead, lactoferrin is an iron binding protein and has a broad spectrum of antimicrobial properties. Its bacteriostatic effect is thought to be due to its ability to sequester environmental iron, because bacteria like *E. coli* secrete chelators to enhance iron uptake.

Thus, healthy individuals on a varied diet benefit from the presence of bioactive peptides that help maintain optimal nervous, immune and digestive systems [97].

Legumes

Legumes are the dried seeds of the *Leguminosae* family: beans, broad beans, lentils, chickpeas and peas. They are vegetables with high protein levels, about 20%, similar to meat. The protein quality is moderate but is higher than that of the cereals that complement them. Digestiblity is poor (particularly for beans) because the proteic fractions are resistant to proteolysis, and because protease inhibitors, lectins and phenolic compounds are present. Fortunately, cooking inactivates protease inhibitors and lectins, but only well cooked legumes are a good source of nutrients. Lipids, mostly PUFA, comprise about 6% by weight in chickpeas, in the other legumes the lipid values are even lower. Dietary fiber in all legumes is notably high, but it is soluble, particularly in beans. All legumes contain vitamins B1, B2, niacin and folates, iron, calcium and zinc, but phytic acid binds the minerals and reduces their bioavailability.

Virgin Olive Oil and Vegetable Oils

The source of the MUFA in MD (about 20% of energy) is mainly olive oil, a culinary dressing. The composition of virgin olive oil, in terms of fatty acid percentage is: 72 oleic, 11 palmitic, 8 linoleic, 1 linolenic, 2 stearic. Olive oil is also a good source of vitamin E, 22.4 mg/100 mL.

The MD is associated with a lower incidence of certain types of cancer, including breast cancer, as well as CHD, a benefit ascribed to the high consumption of extra-virgin olive oil, rich in antioxidants and bioactive compounds. A major phenolic compound in extra-virgin olive oil is oleocanthal, which is known to have anti-inflammatory properties and to contribute to extra-virgin olive oil's sensory characteristics like bitterness. At least 30 phenolic compounds, such oleuropein, oleocanthal, hydroxytyrosol and tyrosol, are found in olive oil, and these act as strong antioxidants, radical scavengers and NSAI- like drugs (Non-steroidal anti-inflammatory drugs).

The n-6 PUFAs can be found in vegetable oils and, in small amounts, in breast milk.

Fish

The MD suggests a moderate to high fish consumption, and it is believed, from observational evidence, that this dietary factor reduces the risk of CHD. There is, however, still the question of whether the benefits are due entirely to the n-3, or long-chain n-3 fatty acids such as docosahexaenoic acid (DHA) and eicosapentaenoic (EPA) and/or other nutrients in fish [98]. It has been reported that marine n-3 PUFAs have anti-atherosclerotic, antithrombotic, anti-arrhythmic and anti-inflammatory effects, all of which might explain the possible beneficial effect on acute coronary syndrome. Humans can biosynthesize EPA (20:5 n-3) and DHA (22:6 n-3) from the parent essential fatty acid alpha-linolenic acid (ALA; 18:3 n-3). However, the low conversion rates of ALA to EPA, particularly DHA, means that the ALA dietary intake must be relatively high and the intake of LA, a metabolic competitor for the biosynthetic pathway, must be low to meet the body's needs for longer chain derivatives. In any case it is not the fish that synthesizes most of these compounds in their tissues: they come from the single-cell marine organisms consumed by fish and shellfish. EPA and DHA are found in fish that live in cold, deep seas [99], while n-3 PUFAs are found in marine algae and the fish oil of tuna, mackerel, herring, salmon and sardines; they also occur naturally in human breast milk.

Nuts

Nuts, nutrient-dense foods with complex matrices, are rich in unsaturated fatty acids and other bioactive compounds such as L-arginine, fiber, minerals, tocopherols, phytosterols and polyphenols. This unique composition of nuts makes them very beneficial for cardiac health. Indeed, epidemiologic studies have revealed that the consumption of nuts leads to reduced coronary disease in men and women, and diabetes in women. There is also some evidence that nuts have a beneficial effect on hypertension and inflammation. Furthermore, it has been shown that nut intake has a cholesterol-lowering effect, beneficial effects on oxidative stress, inflammation and vascular reactivity, and that blood pressure, visceral adiposity and glycemic control can be positively influenced. All these benefits can be achieved by frequent nut consumption, and there is no evidence of undue weight gain [100].

Surprisingly, the cholesterol-lowering effect of nuts was found to be greater than predicted on the basis of the amount and nature of consumed fat, suggesting the presence in nuts of other bioactive components, i.e. polyphenols [101].

Fat bioavailability from nuts could be a factor in the observed hypolipidemic effect. Indeed, the cell wall's physico-chemical structure within the food source and interactions with the lumen of the gastrointestinal tract are important factors that influence nutrient bioavailability. In humans, lipid bioavailability was evaluated by Ellis et al. [102].

Pistachios – The pistachio tree, of which the fruit/seed has both a high nutritional value and a long shelf-life, is now quite widespread throughout the Mediterranean. The key nutrients and phytochemicals of 100 g of seed are as follows: 564 kcal, 44.8 g of total lipids (23.6 g MUFA, 13.4 g PUFA, 5.3 g saturated fats), 20.8 g of proteins, 9.9 g of dietary fiber, 1005 mg of K, 112 mg of Mg, 13 μg of vitamin K, 2.5 mg of vitamin E (α-tocopherol) and 1658 mg of total phenols. The seed's serving size is about 30 g (1 ounce) net weight i.e. without the shell.

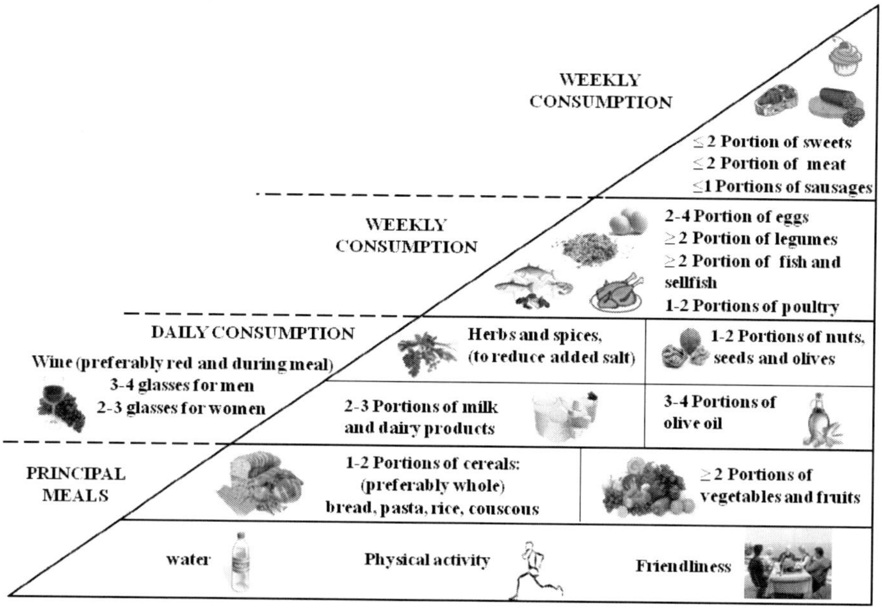

Figure 1. The Italian Mediterranean Diet pyramid. The present figure represents the dietary pattern recommended to Italian population according to the Mediterranean Diet. The schematic presentation summarizes which type of food is to consume every day at principal meals and which is to consume weekly.

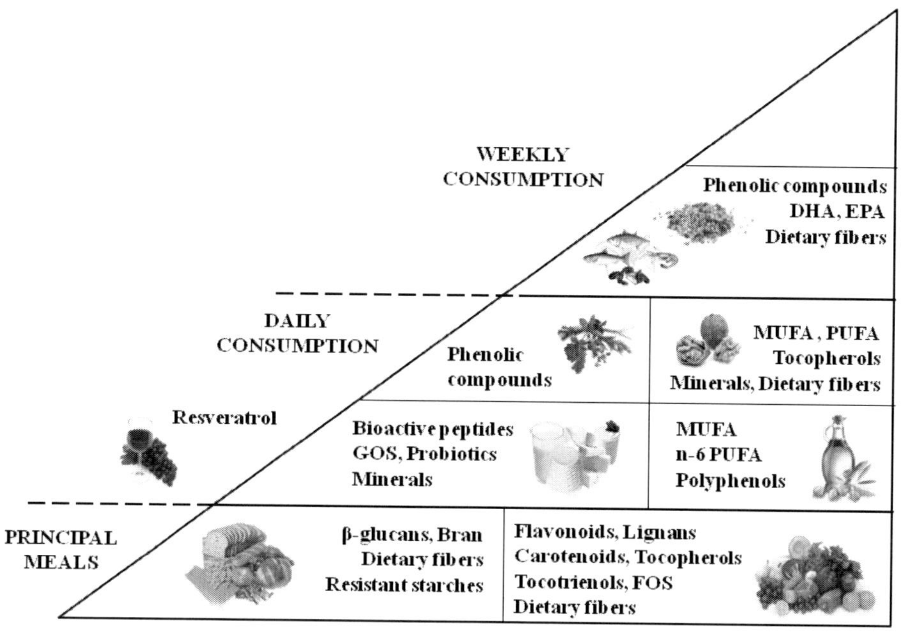

Figure 2. Functional foods and nutraceuticals present in the Mediterranean Diet. The present figure shows the same schematic subdivision of the dietary pattern characteristic of the Italian Mediterranean Diet but substituting the different type of food in each box with the bioactive compounds contained herein.

In a heart-healthy diet the seeds, consumed in moderation, help increase the PUFA and MUFA intake of consumers [103]; oleic and linolenic acids account for about 88% total lipids. Pistachios have lower fat and caloric levels and higher levels of potassium, vitamins K and E, and total phenols than almonds and walnuts [104].

Almonds – The nutrient composition of almonds is for 100 g: 585 kcal, 50.8 g of total lipids (31.7 MUFA, 12.5 PUFA, 3.9 g saturated fats), 21.1 g of proteins, 11.6 of dietary fiber, 693 mg of K, 275 mg of Mg, 25 mg of vitamin E (α-tocopherol), 423 mg of total phenols. There is a favorable shift in a diet's fatty acid profile when almonds are substituted for foods high in saturated fat or carbohydrates, the major fatty acids being oleic acid and linoleic acid that account for 91-94% of total lipids [105]. The serving size of almonds is about 30 g (1 ounce) net weight i.e. without the shell.

Walnuts – The nutrients and phytochemicals for 100 g of walnuts is: 652 kcal, 65.2 g total lipids (8.8 g MUFA, 47.2 g PUFA, 6.0 g of saturated fats), 15 g proteins, 6.6 g dietary fiber, 440 mg K, 158 g Mg, 2.8 μg vitamin K, 0.7mg vitamin E (α-tocopherol), 1552 mg total phenols. Of all the nuts, walnuts have the highest weight % of PUFA, and also the highest % 18:2 (n-6), and the highest % 18:3 (n-3), while the amount of saturated fatty acid is quite low, ranging from 4-15% [101].

Role of Physical Activity in Promoting Health

One's status of health is strongly influenced by hereditary and life-style, particularly by appropriate physical activity and a high-quality diet. A key factor in preventing the development of chronic disease is the maintenance of healthy body weight. Proper physical activity certainly improves one's health in that it helps prevent excessive weight gain, but other factors of health-related fitness can also be cardiovascular-respiratory fitness, adequate muscular strength and endurance, and sufficient flexibility. Physical activity can be either unstructured or structured. Unstructured physical activity is what we do in our everyday life - walking, climbing stairs, cycling, dancing, gardening, yard work, and the various domestic and occupational activities associated with our homes. Structured physical activity (or exercise) is a planned program of physical activities designed to improve physical fitness, including heart-related fitness. Exercise has become an increasingly important means of helping prevent, and even of treating, chronic diseases that afflict developed societies, including coronary artery disease, stroke, hypertension, cancer, diabetes, arthritis, osteoporosis, chronic lung disease and obesity. Indeed, some physicians indicate that exercise is the best medicine of all because it offers such an array of health benefits.

It is important to remember that physical activity does not need to be strenuous to achieve health benefits. Children, adolescents, and men and women of all ages can benefit from a moderate amount of daily physical activity. The benefits of moderate activity may be obtained in longer sessions of moderate intense activities (such as 40 minutes of walking) or in shorter sessions of somewhat more strenuous activities (such 15-20 minutes of running). You should try to average 30 minutes of moderate exercise per day most, and preferably all, days of the week. You may accumulate 30 minutes per days in several sessions, such as three 10-minute brisk walks interspersed throughout the day. Some examples of moderate amounts of physical activity are presented in Table 2.

Table 2. Some examples of moderate amounts of physical activity

Washing windows or floors for 45-60 minutes
Playing various team sports for 45 minutes
Gardening for 30-45 minutes
Bicycling 5 miles (8 km) in 30 minutes
Dancing fast for 30 minutes
Walking 2 miles (3 km) in 30 minutes
Bicycling 4 miles (6.5 km) in 15 minutes
Running 1.5 miles (2.5 km) in 15 minutes
Stair walking for 15 minutes

A moderate amount of physical activity is roughly equivalent to physical activity that uses 150 Calories per day, or 1,000 Calories per week. Note that exercising at lower intensity levels requires more time than exercising at higher intensity levels.

CONCLUSION

This chapter focuses on the MD, specifically the Italian MD, as a recognized dietary pattern able to allow the intakes of all the bioactive compounds known to be associated to positive outcomes for human health. The MD has become a subject of intense studies with the work of Keys [1], known as the Seven Country Studies, but it was with the successive publications as reviewed in Sofi 2009 [106] that the connection with the clinical benefits became more and more evident. The reason of this connection is to be found in the specific choice of foods as well as in the appropriate life habits as a regular physical activity together with the friendliness accompanying the meals. The prevalence in the MD of vegetables and fruits, of cereals and dairy products, of herbs, spices, legumes, nuts, seeds and the correspondent reduction in the consume of red meats, sausages and eggs are key factors responsible of the goodness of this dietary pattern [107], in fact the bioactive compounds or nutraceuticals are largely contained in the food at the base of the MD pyramid, that is food to be consumed daily or with a higher weekly frequency, while at the top of the pyramid their presence is low or absent, one more reason to consume those food with moderation and occasionally. Though MD comprises the life and food habits of all the countries of the Mediterranean basin (Italy, Greece, France, Spain, North Africa, East Basin) some differences inside each specific country foods are evident [106], but the positive outcomes are still present. This statement substantiates the importance of the contemporary presence of all the indicated nutrients in the daily meals to get the above mentioned benefits.

All the studies here mentioned and the important outcomes pointed out has validated the decision to name MD as "intangible cultural heritage by UNESCO".

REFERENCES

[1] Keys, A., Menotti, A., Karvonen, M. J., Aravanis, C., *et al.*, The diet and 15-year death rate in the seven countries study. *Am. J. Epidemiol.* 1986, *124*, 903-915.

[2] Manach, C., Morand, C., Gil-Izquierdo, A., Bouteloup-Demange, C., Remesy, C., Bioavailability in humans of the flavanones hesperidin and narirutin after the ingestion of two doses of orange juice. *Eur. J. Clin. Nutr.* 2003, *57*, 235-242.

[3] Borriello, A., Cucciolla, V., Della Ragione, F., Galletti, P., Dietary polyphenols: focus on resveratrol, a promising agent in the prevention of cardiovascular diseases and control of glucose homeostasis. *Nutr. Metab. Cardiovasc. Dis.* 2010, *20*, 618-625.

[4] Manach, C., Williamson, G., Morand, C., Scalbert, A., Remesy, C., Bioavailability and bioefficacy of polyphenols in humans. I. Review of 97 bioavailability studies. *Am. J. Clin. Nutr.* 2005, *81*, 230S-242S.

[5] Williamson, G., Manach, C., Bioavailability and bioefficacy of polyphenols in humans. II. Review of 93 intervention studies. *Am. J. Clin. Nutr.* 2005, *81*, 243S-255S.

[6] Sies, H., Stahl, W., Sundquist, A. R., Antioxidant functions of vitamins. Vitamins E and C, beta-carotene, and other carotenoids. *Ann. N. Y. Acad. Sci.* 1992, *669*, 7-20.

[7] van Het Hof, K. H., West, C. E., Weststrate, J. A., Hautvast, J. G., Dietary factors that affect the bioavailability of carotenoids. *J. Nutr.* 2000, *130*, 503-506.

[8] Fernández-García, E., Carvajal-Lérida, I., Jarén-Galán, M., Garrido-Fernández, J., *et al.*, Carotenoids bioavailability from foods: From plant pigments to efficient biological activities. *Food Research International* 2012, *46*, 438-450.

[9] Palozza, P., Catalano, A., Simone, R., Cittadini, A., Lycopene as a guardian of redox signalling. *Acta Biochimica Polonica* 2012, *59*, 21-25.

[10] Aggarwal, B. B., Sundaram, C., Prasad, S., Kannappan, R., Tocotrienols, the vitamin E of the 21st century: its potential against cancer and other chronic diseases. *Biochem. Pharmacol.* 2010, *80*, 1613-1631.

[11] Cook-Mills, J. M., McCary, C. A., Isoforms of vitamin E differentially regulate inflammation. *Endocr. Metab. Immune Disord. Drug Targets* 2010, *10*, 348-366.

[12] Sylvester, P. W., Kaddoumi, A., Nazzal, S., El Sayed, K. A., The value of tocotrienols in the prevention and treatment of cancer. *J. Am. Coll. Nutr.* 2010, *29*, 324S-333S.

[13] Nag, S. A., Qin, J. J., Wang, W., Wang, M. H., *et al.*, Ginsenosides as Anticancer Agents: In vitro and in vivo Activities, Structure-Activity Relationships, and Molecular Mechanisms of Action. *Front Pharmacol.* 2012, *3*, 25.

[14] Berg, A., Konig, D., Deibert, P., Grathwohl, D., *et al.*, Effect of an oat bran enriched diet on the atherogenic lipid profile in patients with an increased coronary heart disease risk. A controlled randomized lifestyle intervention study. *Ann. Nutr. Metab.* 2003, *47*, 306-311.

[15] Dongowski, G., Huth, M., Gebhardt, E., Flamme, W., Dietary fiber-rich barley products beneficially affect the intestinal tract of rats. *J. Nutr.* 2002, *132*, 3704-3714.

[16] Odes, H. S., Lazovski, H., Stern, I., Madar, Z., Fiber-enriched cereal for constipation and for hypercholesterolemia. *Harefuah* 1993, *125*, 136-138, 192.

[17] Delaney, B., Carlson, T., Zheng, G. H., Hess, R., *et al.*, Repeated dose oral toxicological evaluation of concentrated barley beta-glucan in CD-1 mice including a recovery phase. *Food Chem. Toxicol.* 2003, *41*, 1089-1102.

[18] Wisker, E., Daniel, M., Rave, G., Feldheim, W., Short-chain fatty acids produced in vitro from fibre residues obtained from mixed diets containing different breads and in human faeces during the ingestion of the diets. *Br. J. Nutr.* 2000, *84*, 31-37.

[19] Granfeldt, Y., Nyberg, L., Bjorck, I., Muesli with 4 g oat beta-glucans lowers glucose and insulin responses after a bread meal in healthy subjects. *Eur. J. Clin. Nutr.* 2008, *62*, 600-607.
[20] Drzikova, B., Dongowski, G., Gebhardt, E., Dietary fibre-rich oat-based products affect serum lipids, microbiota, formation of short-chain fatty acids and steroids in rats. *Br. J. Nutr.* 2005, *94*, 1012-1025.
[21] Choi, J. S., Kim, H., Jung, M. H., Hong, S., Song, J., Consumption of barley beta-glucan ameliorates fatty liver and insulin resistance in mice fed a high-fat diet. *Mol. Nutr. Food Res.* 2010, *54*, 1004-1013.
[22] Brown, L., Rosner, B., Willett, W. W., Sacks, F. M., Cholesterol-lowering effects of dietary fiber: a meta-analysis. *Am. J. Clin. Nutr.* 1999, *69*, 30-42.
[23] Triplehorn, C., Millard, P. S., A rice-based diet with green banana or pectin reduced diarrhea in infants better than a rice-alone diet. *ACP J. Club* 2002, *136*, 67.
[24] Olano-Martin, E., Gibson, G. R., Rastell, R. A., Comparison of the in vitro bifidogenic properties of pectins and pectic-oligosaccharides. *J. Appl. Microbiol.* 2002, *93*,505-511.
[25] Qureshi, A. A., Sami, S. A., Khan, F. A., Effects of stabilized rice bran, its soluble and fiber fractions on blood glucose levels and serum lipid parameters in humans with diabetes mellitus Types I and II. *J. Nutr. Biochem.* 2002, *13*, 175-187.
[26] Behall, K. M., Scholfield, D. J., Hallfrisch, J. G., Liljeberg-Elmstahl, H. G., Consumption of both resistant starch and beta-glucan improves postprandial plasma glucose and insulin in women. *Diabetes Care* 2006, *29*, 976-981.
[27] Lattimer, J. M., Haub, M. D., Effects of dietary fiber and its components on metabolic health. *Nutrients* 2010, *2*, 1266-1289.
[28] Astrup, A., Meinert Larsen, T., Harper, A., Atkins and other low-carbohydrate diets: hoax or an effective tool for weight loss? *Lancet* 2004, *364*, 897-899.
[29] Santesso, N., Akl, E. A., Bianchi, M., Mente, A., *et al.*, Effects of higher- versus lower-protein diets on health outcomes: a systematic review and meta-analysis. *Eur. J. Clin. Nutr.* 2012, *66*, 780-788.
[30] Clifton, P. M., Bastiaans, K., Keogh, J. B., High protein diets decrease total and abdominal fat and improve CVD risk profile in overweight and obese men and women with elevated triacylglycerol. *Nutr. Metab. Cardiovasc. Dis.* 2009, *19*, 548-554.
[31] Bernstein, A. M., Sun, Q., Hu, F. B., Stampfer, M. J., *et al.*, Major dietary protein sources and risk of coronary heart disease in women. *Circulation* 2010, *122*, 876-883.
[32] Bernstein, A. M., Pan, A., Rexrode, K. M., Stampfer, M., *et al.*, Dietary protein sources and the risk of stroke in men and women. *Stroke* 2012, *43*, 637-644.
[33] Bravata, D. M., Sanders, L., Huang, J., Krumholz, H. M., *et al.*, Efficacy and safety of low-carbohydrate diets: a systematic review. *JAMA* 2003, *289*, 1837-1850.
[34] Samaha, F. F., Iqbal, N., Seshadri, P., Chicano, K. L., *et al.*, A low-carbohydrate as compared with a low-fat diet in severe obesity. *N. Engl. J. Med.* 2003, *348*, 2074-2081.
[35] Lagiou, P., Sandin, S., Lof, M., Trichopoulos, D., *et al.*, Low carbohydrate-high protein diet and incidence of cardiovascular diseases in Swedish women: prospective cohort study. *BMJ* 2012, *344*, e4026.
[36] Riemersma, R. A., Wood, D. A., Butler, S., Elton, R. A., *et al.*, Linoleic acid content in adipose tissue and coronary heart disease. *Br. Med. J. (Clin. Res. Ed.)* 1986, *292*, 1423-1427.

[37] Valek, J., Hammer, J., Kohout, M., Grafnetter, D., *et al.*, Serum linoleic acid and cardiovascular death in postinfarction middle-aged men. *Atherosclerosis* 1985, *54*, 111-118.

[38] Simpson, H. C., Barker, K., Carter, R. D., Cassels, E., Mann, J. I., Low dietary intake of linoleic acid predisposes to myocardial infarction. *Br. Med. J. (Clin. Res. Ed.)* 1982, *285*, 683-684.

[39] Hegsted, D. M., Ausman, L. M., Diet, alcohol and coronary heart disease in men. *J. Nutr.* 1988, *118*, 1184-1189.

[40] Baylin, A., Kabagambe, E. K., Ascherio, A., Spiegelman, D., Campos, H., Adipose tissue alpha-linolenic acid and nonfatal acute myocardial infarction in Costa Rica. *Circulation* 2003, *107*, 1586-1591.

[41] Djousse, L., Folsom, A. R., Province, M. A., Hunt, S. C., Ellison, R. C., Dietary linolenic acid and carotid atherosclerosis: the National Heart, Lung, and Blood Institute Family Heart Study. *Am. J. Clin. Nutr.* 2003, *77*, 819-825.

[42] Wijendran, V., Hayes, K. C., Dietary n-6 and n-3 fatty acid balance and cardiovascular health. *Annu. Rev. Nutr.* 2004, *24*, 597-615.

[43] Wall, R., Ross, R. P., Fitzgerald, G. F., Stanton, C., Fatty acids from fish: the anti-inflammatory potential of long-chain omega-3 fatty acids. *Nutr. Rev.* 2010, *68*,280-289.

[44] Gibson, G. R., Probert, H. M., Loo, J. V., Rastall, R. A., Roberfroid, M. B., Dietary modulation of the human colonic microbiota: updating the concept of prebiotics. *Nutr. Res. Rev.* 2004, *17*, 259-275.

[45] Snart, J., Bibiloni, R., Grayson, T., Lay, C., *et al.*, Supplementation of the diet with high-viscosity beta-glucan results in enrichment for lactobacilli in the rat cecum. *Appl. Environ. Microbiol.* 2006, *72*, 1925-1931.

[46] Arslanoglu, S., Moro, G. E., Schmitt, J., Tandoi, L., *et al.*, Early dietary intervention with a mixture of prebiotic oligosaccharides reduces the incidence of allergic manifestations and infections during the first two years of life. *J. Nutr.* 2008, *138*, 1091-1095.

[47] Bruzzese, E., Volpicelli, M., Squeglia, V., Bruzzese, D., *et al.*, A formula containing galacto- and fructo-oligosaccharides prevents intestinal and extra-intestinal infections: an observational study. *Clin. Nutr.* 2009, *28*, 156-161.

[48] Arslanoglu, S., Moro, G. E., Boehm, G., Early supplementation of prebiotic oligosaccharides protects formula-fed infants against infections during the first 6 months of life. *J. Nutr.* 2007, *137*, 2420-2424.

[49] Tschernia, A., Moore, N., Abi-Hanna, A., Yolken, R., *et al.*, Effects of long-term consumption of a weaning food supplemented with oligofructose, a prebiotic, on general infant health status. *Journal of Pediatric Gastroenterology and Nutrition* 1999, *29*, 503.

[50] Searle, L. E., Best, A., Nunez, A., Salguero, F. J., *et al.*, A mixture containing galactooligosaccharide, produced by the enzymic activity of Bifidobacterium bifidum, reduces Salmonella enterica serovar Typhimurium infection in mice. *J. Med. Microbiol.* 2009, *58*, 37-48.

[51] Shoaf, K., Mulvey, G. L., Armstrong, G. D., Hutkins, R. W., Prebiotic galactooligosaccharides reduce adherence of enteropathogenic Escherichia coli to tissue culture cells. *Infect. Immun.* 2006, *74*, 6920-6928.

[52] Guilloteau, P., Martin, L., Eeckhaut, V., Ducatelle, R., *et al.*, From the gut to the peripheral tissues: the multiple effects of butyrate. *Nutr. Res. Rev.* 2010, *23*, 366-384.

[53] Arbeitsgruppe, Probiotische, Mikroorganismen, in, Lebensmitteln, Bundesinstitut für gesundheitlichen Verbraucherschutz und Veterinärmedizin, Berlin 2000, pp. 191-195.

[54] de Vrese, M., Schrezenmeir, J., Probiotics, prebiotics, and synbiotics. *Adv. Biochem. Eng. Biotechnol.* 2008, *111*, 1-66.

[55] Allen, S. J., Okoko, B., Martinez, E., Gregorio, G., Dans, L. F., Probiotics for treating infectious diarrhoea. *Cochrane Database Syst. Rev.* 2004, CD003048.

[56] Huang, J. S., Bousvaros, A., Lee, J. W., Diaz, A., Davidson, E. J., Efficacy of probiotic use in acute diarrhea in children: a meta-analysis. *Dig. Dis. Sci.* 2002, *47*, 2625-2634.

[57] Chandra, R. K., Effect of *Lactobacillus* on the incidence and severity of acute rotavirus diarrhoea in infants. A prospective placebo-controlled double-blind study. *Nutrition Research* 2002, *22*, 65-69.

[58] de Roos, N. M., Katan, M. B., Effects of probiotic bacteria on diarrhea, lipid metabolism, and carcinogenesis: a review of papers published between 1988 and 1998. *Am. J. Clin. Nutr.* 2000, *71*, 405-411.

[59] Aso, Y., Akaza, H., Kotake, T., Tsukamoto, T., *et al.*, Preventive effect of a Lactobacillus casei preparation on the recurrence of superficial bladder cancer in a double-blind trial. The BLP Study Group. *Eur. Urol.* 1995, *27*, 104-109.

[60] Oatley, J. T., Rarick, M. D., Ji, G. E., Linz, J. E., Binding of aflatoxin B1 to bifidobacteria in vitro. *J. Food Prot.* 2000, *63*, 1133-1136.

[61] Fric, P., Zavoral, M., The effect of non-pathogenic Escherichia coli in symptomatic uncomplicated diverticular disease of the colon. *Eur. J. Gastroenterol. Hepatol.* 2003, *15*, 313-315.

[62] Ishikawa, H., Akedo, I., Umesaki, Y., Tanaka, R., *et al.*, Randomized controlled trial of the effect of bifidobacteria-fermented milk on ulcerative colitis. *J. Am. Coll. Nutr.* 2003, *22*, 56-63.

[63] Peluso, I., Fina, D., Caruso, R., Stolfi, C., *et al.*, Lactobacillus paracasei subsp. paracasei B21060 suppresses human T-cell proliferation. *Infect. Immun.* 2007, *75*, 1730-1737.

[64] Isolauri, E., Arvola, T., Sutas, Y., Moilanen, E., Salminen, S., Probiotics in the management of atopic eczema. *Clin. Exp. Allergy* 2000, *30*, 1604-1610.

[65] Rosenfeldt, V., Benfeldt, E., Nielsen, S. D., Michaelsen, K. F., *et al.*, Effect of probiotic Lactobacillus strains in children with atopic dermatitis. *J. Allergy Clin. Immunol.* 2003, *111*, 389-395.

[66] de Vrese, M., Rautenberg, P., Laue, C., Koopmans, M., *et al.*, Probiotic bacteria stimulate virus-specific neutralizing antibodies following a booster polio vaccination. *Eur. J. Nutr.* 2005, *44*, 406-413.

[67] Turchet, P., Laurenzano, M., Auboiron, S., Antoine, J. M., Effect of fermented milk containing the probiotic Lactobacillus casei DN-114001 on winter infections in free-living elderly subjects: a randomised, controlled pilot study. *J. Nutr. Health Aging* 2003, *7*, 75-77.

[68] Caimi, G., Carollo, C., Lo Presti, R., Wine and endothelial function. *Drugs Exp. Clin. Res.* 2003, *29*, 235-242.

[69] Baur, J. A., Pearson, K. J., Price, N. L., Jamieson, H. A., *et al.*, Resveratrol improves health and survival of mice on a high-calorie diet. *Nature* 2006, *444*, 337-342.

[70] Barger, J. L., Kayo, T., Vann, J. M., Arias, E. B., *et al.*, A low dose of dietary resveratrol partially mimics caloric restriction and retards aging parameters in mice. *PLoS One* 2008, *3*, e2264.

[71] Viuda-Martos, M., Ruiz-Navajas, Y., Fernandez-Lopez, J., Perez-Alvarez, J. A., Spices as functional foods. *Crit. Rev. Food Sci. Nutr.* 2011, *51*, 13-28.

[72] Kim, J. Y., Kwon, O., Culinary plants and their potential impact on metabolic overload. *Ann. N. Y. Acad. Sci.* 2011, *1229*, 133-139.

[73] Tapsell, L. C., Hemphill, I., Cobiac, L., Patch, C. S., *et al.*, Health benefits of herbs and spices: the past, the present, the future. *Med. J. Aust.* 2006, *185*, S4-24.

[74] Wirfalt, E., McTaggart, A., Pala, V., Gullberg, B., *et al.*, Food sources of carbohydrates in a European cohort of adults. *Public Health Nutr* 2002, *5*, 1197-1215.

[75] Mellen, P. B., Walsh, T. F., Herrington, D. M., Whole grain intake and cardiovascular disease: a meta-analysis. *Nutr. Metab. Cardiovasc. Dis.* 2008, *18*, 283-290.

[76] Nettleton, J. A., McKeown, N. M., Kanoni, S., Lemaitre, R. N., *et al.*, Interactions of dietary whole-grain intake with fasting glucose- and insulin-related genetic loci in individuals of European descent: a meta-analysis of 14 cohort studies. *Diabetes Care* 2010, *33*, 2684-2691.

[77] Okarter, N., Liu, R. H., Health benefits of whole grain phytochemicals. *Crit. Rev. Food Sci. Nutr.* 2010, *50*, 193-208.

[78] Adom, K. K., Sorrells, M. E., Liu, R. H., Phytochemicals and antioxidant activity of milled fractions of different wheat varieties. *J. Agric. Food Chem.* 2005, *53*, 2297-2306.

[79] Slavin, J., Whole grains and human health. *Nutr. Res. Rev.* 2004, *17*, 99-110.

[80] Harland, J. I., Garton, L. E., Whole-grain intake as a marker of healthy body weight and adiposity. *Public Health Nutr.* 2008, *11*, 554-563.

[81] Jonnalagadda, S. S., Harnack, L., Liu, R. H., McKeown, N., *et al.*, Putting the whole grain puzzle together: health benefits associated with whole grains--summary of American Society for Nutrition 2010 Satellite Symposium. *J. Nutr.* 2011, *141*, 1011S-1022S.

[82] Seal, C. J., Brownlee, I. A., Whole Grains and Health, Evidence from Observational and Intervention Studies. *Cereal Chemistry* 2010, *87*, 167-174.

[83] Wang, L., Gaziano, J. M., Liu, S., Manson, J. E., *et al.*, Whole- and refined-grain intakes and the risk of hypertension in women. *Am. J. Clin. Nutr.* 2007, *86*, 472-479.

[84] Tucker, L. A., Thomas, K. S., Increasing total fiber intake reduces risk of weight and fat gains in women. *J. Nutr.* 2009, *139*, 576-581.

[85] Park, Y., Brinton, L. A., Subar, A. F., Hollenbeck, A., Schatzkin, A., *Am. J. Clin. Nutr.*, United States 2009, pp. 664-671.

[86] Streppel, M. T., Ocke, M. C., Boshuizen, H. C., Kok, F. J., Kromhout, D., Dietary fiber intake in relation to coronary heart disease and all-cause mortality over 40 y: the Zutphen Study. *Am. J. Clin. Nutr.* 2008, *88*, 1119-1125.

[87] Schatzkin, A., Park, Y., Leitzmann, M. F., Hollenbeck, A. R., Cross, A. J., Prospective study of dietary fiber, whole grain foods, and small intestinal cancer. *Gastroenterology* 2008, *135*, 1163-1167.

[88] Liu, S., Stampfer, M. J., Hu, F. B., Giovannucci, E., *et al.*, Whole-grain consumption and risk of coronary heart disease: results from the Nurses' Health Study. *Am. J. Clin. Nutr.* 1999, *70*, 412-419.

[89] Ferguson, L. R., Chavan, R. R., Harris, P. J., Changing concepts of dietary fiber: implications for carcinogenesis. *Nutr. Cancer* 2001, *39*, 155-169.

[90] Weickert, M. O., Mohlig, M., Schofl, C., Arafat, A. M., *et al.*, Cereal fiber improves whole-body insulin sensitivity in overweight and obese women. *Diabetes Care* 2006, *29*, 775-780.

[91] Keenan, H. A., Doria, A., Aiello, L. P., King, G. L., Positivity of C-peptide, GADA and IA2 antibodies in type 1 diabetic patients with extreme duration. *Diabetes* 2006,*55*,A65.

[92] INRAN, Tabelle di composizione degli alimenti, 2000, EDRA - Medical Publishing and New Media.

[93] de Leeuw, P. W., van der Zander, K., Kroon, A. A., Rennenberg, R. M., Koning, M. M., Dose-dependent lowering of blood pressure by dairy peptides in mildly hypertensive subjects. *Blood Press* 2009, *18*, 44-50.

[94] Meisel, H., Bioactive peptides from milk proteins: a perspective for consumers and producers. *Aust. J. Dairy Technol.* 2001, *56*, 83-93.

[95] Ferraretto, A., Fiorilli, A., in: Avigliano, L., Rossi, L. (Eds.), *Biochemical aspects of human nutrition*, Transworld Research Network, Kerala India 2010, pp. 69-86.

[96] Fiorilli, A., Perego, S., Ferraretto, A., in: Ventimiglia, A. M., Birkenhäger, J. M. (Eds.), *Casein: production, uses and health effects*, Nova Science Publishers, Inc., NY 2011, pp. 83-100.

[97] Nagpal, R., Behare, P., Rana, R., Kumar, A., *et al.*, Bioactive peptides derived from milk proteins and their health beneficial potentials: an update. *Food Funct.* 2011, *2*, 18-27.

[98] Eckel, R. H., The fish oil story remains fishy. *Circulation* 2010, *122*, 2110-2112.

[99] Berge, J. P., Barnathan, G., Fatty acids from lipids of marine organisms: molecular biodiversity, roles as biomarkers, biologically active compounds, and economical aspects. *Adv. Biochem. Eng. Biotechnol.* 2005, *96*, 49-125.

[100] Ros, E., Tapsell, L. C., Sabate, J., Nuts and berries for heart health. *Curr. Atheroscler. Rep.* 2010, *12*, 397-406.

[101] Vinson, J. A., Cai, Y., Nuts, especially walnuts, have both antioxidant quantity and efficacy and exhibit significant potential health benefits. *Food Funct.* 2012, *3*, 134-140.

[102] Ellis, P. R., Kendall, C. W., Ren, Y., Parker, C., *et al.*, Role of cell walls in the bioaccessibility of lipids in almond seeds. *Am. J. Clin. Nutr.* 2004, *80*, 604-613.

[103] Dreher, M. L., Pistachio nuts: composition and potential health benefits. *Nutr. Rev.* 2012, *70*, 234-240.

[104] *USDA*, N*ational*, N*utrient*, *Database*, *et al.*, in: US Department of Agriculture, A. R. S. (Ed.), Agricultural Research Service, US Dept of Agriculture, Beltsville, MD 2011.

[105] Berryman, C. E., Preston, A. G., Karmally, W., Deckelbaum, R. J., Kris-Etherton, P. M., Effects of almond consumption on the reduction of LDL-cholesterol: a discussion of potential mechanisms and future research directions. *Nutr. Rev.* 2011, *69*, 171-185.

[106] Sofi, F., The Mediterranean diet revisited: evidence of its effectiveness grows. *Curr. Opin. Cardiol.* 2009, *24*, 442-446.

[107] Saura-Calixto, F., Goni, I., Definition of the Mediterranean diet based on bioactive compounds. *Crit. Rev. Food Sci. Nutr.* 2009, *49*, 145-152.

In: Functional Foods
Editors: Aron Robinson and Dominick Emerson ISBN: 978-1-62417-435-3

Chapter 4

EUROPEAN CONSUMERS ACCEPTANCE OF HEALTHY FOOD PRODUCTS: A REVIEW OF FUNCTIONAL FOODS

***Azzurra Annunziata*[1,*] *and Riccardo Vecchio*[2]**
[1]University of Naples "Parthenope", Naples, Italy
[2]University of Naples Federico II, Portici, Italy

ABSTRACT

In the recent past, Europe has experienced an increase in several chronic diseases linked to dietary and lifestyle habits. In particular, obesity is continuously increasing at an alarming rate all over Europe. As a result healthier food products have rapidly gained important market shares. The food industry has rapidly reacted to this trend by developing a growing variety of new products with health-related claims and images, including functional foods (FF) that are selected by consumers for their health-promoting properties. However, demand for FF within the European Union varies considerably from country to country, mainly due to food traditions and different cultural heritage. This chapter offers an overview of the current FF market situation in Europe and addresses the main cognitive, motivational and attitudinal determinants of consumer acceptance of these foods in different European countries, providing practical insights of the profile of FF consumers. In particular, the major factors that are currently restraining growth of FF in Europe (beyond economic crisis) are highlighted and deeply discussed. As the lack of categorisation (it is still difficult for consumers to distinguish between functional and conventional food products); growing consumer confusion (due to increasing product variety and product labelling, together with the overwhelming amount of general marketing and educational messages on food intake); low awareness of health benefits of functional ingredients; lack of consensus on the level of scientific support and documentation required for specific health claims. The current work could help practitioners in making more effective strategic and tactical marketing decisions, and add some useful information for government bodies interested in designing public health programs.

* azzurra.annunziata@uniparthenope.it.

1. Introduction

In the recent past, Europe has experienced an increase in several chronic diseases linked to dietary and lifestyle factors. In particular, obesity is continuously increasing at an alarming rate all over Europe. According to statistics from the World Health Organization (2007) from 1990 to 2006, obesity levels in Europe tripled on the whole. On average across EU countries, 15.5% of the adult population is obese. As obesity increases the risk of chronic diseases it is estimated that total healthcare costs linked to overweight could increase by as much as 70% between 2007 and 2015 (EUFIC, 2006). In this scenario, consumer health awareness continues to grow together with increasing availability of health information, ageing of populations and increased risk for lifestyle diseases (Kearney, 2010). Indeed European consumers are aware that, together with physical exercise, a proper dietary regime is the most important factor for maintaining a satisfactory state of health (Bech-Larsen and Scholderer, 2007). Therefore the trend in society is to demand healthy food with added health improving benefits (Bleiel, 2010). Demographic trends and socioeconomic changes also make it necessary to have access to foods endowed with more beneficial properties (Sirò *et al.*, 2008). At the same time, increasing of health care costs in most of these countries encourage the development of food products with additional health benefits based on their functional ingredients. As a consequence new technologies have emerged that allow the altering of foods in ways that provide additional health benefits to consumers and healthier food products have rapidly gained important market shares. In this context, functional foods (FF) are a relatively new concept, which has emerged as a result of this increasing focus on, and awareness of, the influence of everyday diet on health (Poulsen, 1999). FF represent certainly one of the most interesting areas of research and innovation in the food industry (Sirò *et al.*, 2008; Jones and Jew, 2007). The concept of FF derives from the realization that specific components of the diet have the capacity to convey benefits beyond those of basic nutrition. FF products are produced both in order to increase the interest in food and health among the public and to facilitate individuals to take responsibility for eating in a healthy way.

Many definitions exist worldwide for FF, but there is no official unanimous accepted description (Kotilainen *et al.* 2006). The European Commission's Concerted Action on Functional Food Science in Europe (FUFOSE), coordinated by ILSI Europe, proposed a working definition of FF: *a food that beneficially affects one or more target functions in the body beyond adequate nutritional effects in a way that is relevant to either an improved state of health and well-being and/or reduction of risk of disease. It is consumed as part of a normal food pattern. It is not a pill, a capsule or any form of dietary supplement.*

The basic features of a FF[1] include the following:

- being a conventional or everyday food,
- being consumed as part of the normal/usual diet,

[1] Functional food can be classified according to several principles, namely the food group it belongs to (e.g. dairy products, beverages, cereal products, confectionary, oils and fats), the diseases it is expected to prevent or alleviate (e.g. diabetes, osteoporosis, colon cancer), its physiological effects (e.g. immunology, digestibility, anti-tumour activity), the category of its specific biologically active ingredients (e.g. minerals, antioxidants, lipids, probiotics), its physico-chemical and organoleptic properties (e.g. colour, solubility, texture), or the processes that are used in its production (e.g. chromatography, encapsulation, freezing) (see among others Juvan et al,. 2005).

- composed of naturally occurring (as opposed to synthetic) components, perhaps in unnatural concentration or present in foods that would not normally supply them,
- having a positive effect on target function(s) beyond nutritive value/basic nutrition,
- may enhance well-being and health and/or reduce the risk of disease or provide health benefit so as to improve the quality of life, including physical, psychological and behavioral performances,
- having an authorized and scientifically based claims.

However, due to the many differences in definitions of FF (see for a complete description, among others: Doyon and Labrecque, 2008; Roberfroid, 2000), market size estimations, within the EU and globally, are not consistent across different studies and reports. Nevertheless, in the recent past a plethora of studies have shown that FF represent a rapidly developing and particularly promising market segment. In Europe, FF sales have increased significantly; currently Germany, France, the United Kingdom and the Netherlands represent the most important countries within the FF market. While many other European markets are experiencing high growth rates (such as Spain).

Nonetheless, demand for FF within the EU varies considerably from country to country mainly due to food traditions and cultural heritage. Moreover, several studies have demonstrated that interest of consumers towards FF in central and northern European states is higher than in Mediterranean countries. Even if, recently, several scholars have indicated that the need for FF is increasingly questioned in Northern European countries, hence yielding the conclusion that consumer acceptance of FF cannot be taken for granted.

Based on these evidence, the present chapter reports the findings of a systematic review that examined published research on European consumer attitudes towards FF.

In particular, the European market of FF is briefly described, subsequently the high demand heterogeneity, linked to the existence of marked regional differences in the perception and willingness to use FF, is presented. Demonstrating that the high heterogeneity stems mainly from socio-demographic differences, the existence of dissimilar dietary habits, the different national policies for the promotion of public health, but also differences related to cultural traditions (Canavari *et al.*, 2007). Furthermore, the main differences among European consumers of FF are highlighted and finally the core strategies for development and marketing of FF are debated. The current review aims to rationalize the vast existing body of evidence on consumers understanding and use FF and identify further interesting research avenues. In addition, gaps in existing research are underlined and critically discussed.

2. Overview of Functional Foods Market

Since no universally accepted definition for FF exists (Kotilainen *et al.*, 2006) typically a food marketed as functional contains added, technologically developed ingredients with a specific health benefit (Niva, 2007). Due to the very ambiguous limits and unclear borderlines of the FF market, estimates of its real value are quite variable and rough. Even so, academic researchers and professionals agree that FF represent a rapidly developing and particularly promising market segment (FAO, 2007; Verbeke, 2005; Menrad, 2003). Currently European consumption levels of FF are limited compared to other traditional consumer countries. As the Japan Ministry of Health Labour and Welfare estimated, in 2007 pro-capite annual expenditure for FF was of 130 US$ in Japan, 70 US$ in the USA and around 50 US$ in Europe.

Consistently, recent data reveal that around 33% of North Americans regularly purchase milk with added supplements or vitamins matched up to only 9% of Europeans; and 26% of North Americans regularly buy bread with added calcium compared to 7% of Europeans (AC Nielsen, 2007).

According to a Datamonitor report (2007) FF market value in Europe reached € 6.4 billion, and the respective market shares of FF in the total food market was estimated to fall into a range of 1-3 percent (Kotilainen *et al.*, 2006). In addition, the same report calculated that in Europe in 2004 8.8% of all new food launched on the market had a nutraceutical[2] claim compared with a percentage of 5.5% in 2001. However, within Europe, the market for FF has developed at different rates in different countries. Allegedly the most important market for FF (including beverages) is the UK with a total value of £785 million in 2010 (Mintel, 2011), followed by Germany, France and the Netherlands (Makinen-Aakula, 2006). These markets have experienced growth rates around 15-20% for many years, slowing robustly after 2008 due to global economic crisis. Nonetheless significant increases in FF sales have been reported in many other European countries (Jago, 2009). Consequently, FF have been developed in virtually all food categories. Recently, the market is dominated by gut health products, in particular probiotics and prebiotics (Jones and Jew, 2007; Alzamora *et al.*, 2005). A European research involving around 6,000 consumers in six countries (UK, Germany, France, Italy, Poland and Portugal) showed that about 38 percent of consumers look to lower cholesterol when consuming FF, roughly the same share cited 'to control blood sugar' and 36 percent 'to reduce weight'.

Taking a closer look to specific functional products we can notice different growth rates for different foods: ranging from 20 to 26 percent for probiotic dairy products (Frost and Sullivan 2003) and around 20 percent for soft drinks.

Quoting the European Commission report on FF, in 2004 on the market there were 385 different products, ranging from dairy foods, beverages, cereals, confectionary and bakery. Even so, the FF market is still characterised by a high level of product failures. During the years almost all companies have been forced to withdraw products. Powerful examples are Nestlé dismissing its functional smoothies, Danone axing its fortified mineral water range and Coca-Cola retreating its 5 Alive functional juice drink.

A rough estimation counts currently around 170 companies in the EU that market at least one FF product, concentrated mainly in Germany and in the UK, followed by Spain and the Netherlands. Leader companies in Europe are Nestlè, Danone, Kellogg's and Unilever, mostly involved in the functional dairy category. While pharmaceuticals companies have often failed the launch of FF[3] (Euromonitor, 2009; Menrad, 2003). Moreover, unlike organic and vegetarian foods, also private labelled FF have had little market success (Organic Monitor, 2009).

[2] The term nutraceutical (coined in 1989 from nutrition and pharmaceutical) is often used as a synonymous of functional food, since currently no clear regulatory distinction has been developed.

[3] Specifically, scholars pointed out pharmaceutical companies' lack of competencies in the optimization of sensory properties of foods, lack of negotiation power in securing retail distribution for the products, and lack of experience with attractive pricing and packaging of foods.

In addition, FF compete in sales with organic, reduced fat, reduced salt, or reduced sugar foods. As a result, to battle in such highly competitive markets, it is important for marketers to use the most effective marketing tools and elaborate valuable messages to communicate to consumers. However, recent experiences show that dissimilar paths are taken by key manufacturers: Danone decided to sell products like Actimel based on strong brand identities, while other producers focus on the properties of functional ingredients and their health benefits, or some companies launch fortified products under existing brand names to broaden consumer appeal.

3. Determinants of Consumer Acceptance of Functional Foods in European Countries

Consumer acceptance has been often identified as the decisive factor in the successful marketing of FF, as a consequence in recent years numerous papers have reported empirical studies based on primary data collection in the European Union. These works have mainly addressed cognitive, motivational and attitudinal determinants of consumer acceptance of FF in different countries. A snapshot of recent European studies on FF consumers is provided in Table 1; these studies vary widely in terms of focus and applied methodologies.

As some recent studies have focused on consumer awareness and acceptance of FF (Stein and Rodríguez-Cerezo, 2008; Bech-Larsen *et al.*, 2001; Moskowitz, Beckley, & Minkus-McKenna, 2004; Niva, 2007; Niva and Makela, 2007; Urala and Lahteenmaki, 2004; van Kleef *et al.*, 2005; Verbeke, 2005), characterization of FF consumers (Szakály *et al.*, 2011; Sparke and Menrad 2009; DeJong *et al.*, 2003) factors motivating consumption of FF (Ares and Gambaro, 2007; Cox and Bastiaans, 2007; Krutulyte *et al.*, 2008), and factors affecting willingness to pay for FF (Hellyer *et al.*, 2012; Marette *et al.*, 2010; Siegrist *et al.*, 2008).

Despite the aforementioned variability of these researches, a review of the literature reveals a number of key factors that influence if and why consumers buy and consume FF, and their general perceptions of FF.

A common result emerging from the literature is that European consumers do not perceive FF as specific products, different from their conventional counterparts; not perceiving FF as members of a particular food category (Siro *et al.*, 2008; Urala and Lahteenmaki, 2003).

Moreover Bech-Larsen and Grunert (2003) claim that European consumers are less inclined to accept FF as a way of making their diet healthier; this may be due to differences in perceptions of what determines healthiness of food and the functional enrichment of foods may have a negative effect on perceived healthiness.

However most of previous studies have demonstrated that cognitive, motivational and attitudinal determinants of consumer acceptance of FF vary considerably in different countries.

Furthermore recent literature also suggests that there may be country differences in acceptance of FF and highlights the importance of conducting specific market research in different states.

Table 1. Recent European studies on functional foods consumers

Research topic	Authors and year of publication	Country	Core findings
General consumer use and acceptance of functional foods	de Jong, Ocké, Branderhorst and Frele 2003	Netherlands	Determinants of FF use depended on the type of product.
	Urala and Lähteenmäki 2003	Finland	Consumers perceive functional products as a member of the general product category such as yoghurt or spread and only secondarily as a FF.
	Urala and Lähteenmäki 2004	Finland	The best predictor for willingness to use FF was the perceived reward.
	Verbeke 2005	Belgium	Belief in the health benefits of FF is the main positive determinant of acceptance.
	Niva and Makela 2007	Finland	Differences in consumer views of FF are mainly linked to the differing roles of food and health in people's lives and the acceptability of modern food technologies.
	Stein and Rodríguez-Cerezo, 2008	Germany, Poland, Spain and the United Kingdom	Among the respondents the term "functional food" was hardly known, but most respondents knew specific products or brands of FF. Generally, correct knowledge of the functionality of ingredients corresponded to a more positive attitude towards FF.
	Krystallis, Maglaras, and Mamalis 2008	Greece	The most important motives of FF purchasing are health enhancement and health risk prevention through appropriate dietary choices.
	Messina, Saba, Turrini, Raats and Lumbers 2008	UK, Denmark, Germany, Poland, Portugal, Spain, Sweden and Italy	Familiarity was the key driver in selecting FF and conventional yogurts.
	Landström, Koivisto Hursti and Magnusson 2009	Sweden	The necessity of FF was justified unless no other lifestyle changes were able to improve a person's state of health.
	Sparke and Menrad 2009	Germany, Poland, Spain, and the United Kingdom	Cross-country comparisons of consumer segments showed distinct shifts of segment distribution in single countries.
	Annunziata and Vecchio 2011	Italy	Perception of healthiness plays a key role in determining shoppers' attitudes toward FF.

Research topic	Authors and year of publication	Country	Core findings
	Szakály, Szente, Polereczki and Szigeti 2011	Hungary	Beliefs, attitudes, subjective norms do not exert great influence on FF purchasing behavior of health conscious consumers.
	Del Giudice and Pascucci 2011	Italy	Different sources of information, knowledge and motivations are key elements in the acceptance of FF.
	Di Pasquale, Adinolfi and Capitanio 2011	Italy	Knowledge and transparency of information appear to be decisive variables in the selection process of FF.
	Markovina, Cacic, Gajdoš Kljusuric and Kovacic 2011	Croatia	The most important FF attributes are taste and price/quality ratio.
	Bitzios, Fraser and Fraser 2011	Netherlands	Simple health statements are prefered compared to, or in addition to, the implied benefits of FF.
Health claims impact on acceptance and use of functional foods	Bech-Larsen and Grunert 2003	Denmark, Finland, USA	Health claims, processing methods, enrichments, product types, are important determinants of consumers' perceptions of the healthiness of functional foods.
	Van Kleef, van Trijp and Luning 2005	Netherlands	Consumer evaluations primarily differ to the extent that health claims are personally relevant in addressing an experienced disease state.
	Verbeke 2005	Belgium	Health benefit belief from FFs emerges as the strongest positive determinant of willingness to compromise on taste.
	Siegrist, Stampfli and Kastenholz 2008	Switzerland	Health claims were most positively evaluated when attached to a product with a positive health image.
	Verbeke, Scholderer and Liisa Lähteenmäki 2009	Belgium	Health claims outperform nutrition claims, and both of these claim types outperform reduction of disease risk claims.
	Marette, Roosen, Blanchemanche and Feinblatt-Mélèze 2010	France	A significant and positive influence of the message linked to the cholesterol reduction exist on willingness to pay for FF.
Product attributes impact on acceptance and use of functional foods	Luckow and Delahunty 2004	Ireland	Consumers preferred the sensory characteristics of conventional compared to FF orange juices.
	Lyly, Roininen, Honkapää, Poutanen and Lähteenmäki 2007	Finland, France and Sweden	Taste of FF strongly affected the willingness to use them.
	Krutulyte, Grunert, Scholderer, Lähteenmäki, Hagemann, Elgaard, Nielsen and Graverholt 2011	Denmark	Perceived carrier–ingredient fit is strongly related to purchase intentions of FF.
	Bonanno 2012	Italy	In the FF yogurt market brand loyalty plays a key role.

3.1. Socio – demographic Factors

A number of demographic background variables - such as gender, age and education - could have some influence on FF acceptance. However, as reported in the literature, the explanatory influence of these variables has been decreasing in developed countries.

Some common results that emerge from recent researches reveal that being female and/or older makes a consumer more likely to have positive attitude towards FF (Pothoulaki and Chryssochoidis, 2009; Verbeke, 2005; Frewer *et al.*, 2003).

Hence female consumers appear as a more promising target group for FF, partly because they show more interest in health in general (Urala 2005; Bogue and Ryan 2000; Childs and Poryzees 1997). Other studies found that FF users have often a higher level of education. Anttolainen and colleagues (2001), DeJong *et al.* (2003) and Pothoulaki and Chryssochoidis (2009), among others, demonstrated that individuals with higher socioeconomic status, particularly high level of education, were more likely to be FF consumers. While, in contrast with this outcome, Verbeke (2005) found that people with a lower level of education and income were more likely to buy FF. Moreover, other research (Verbeke *et al.*, 2009; Urala and Lähteenmäki, 2003) showed that socioeconomic factors such as level of education and health status were insignificant determinants of acceptance and use of FF. Contrasting results have been reported also with respect to the age variable. For example, Poulsen (1999) mentions that older participants in his research (i.e. over 55 years) showed a greater intention to buy FF, while Childs and Poryzees (1997) revealed that the elderly were less intent to buy a food that prevents a disease compared to younger consumers. Verbeke (2006) asserts that middle-aged and elderly consumers are more aware of health issues simply because they, or members of their immediate social environment, are much more likely to be diagnosed with a lifestyle-related disease than are younger consumers. Additionally, according to the findings of Szakály and collegues (2012) there is a significant relationship between lifestyle, health behavior, and the preference for FF. These contradictory findings suggest that profiling FF consumers should not be generalized demographically.

It must be emphasized however, that when considering the influence of gender, age and education, both the type of FF and its claim have to be included. Stewart-Knox et al. (2007) investigated consumer uptake of FF in several European countries (France, Great Britain, Germany, Italy, Poland and Portugal) revealing that younger people, in particular females, seeks for foods to control appetite and body weight, while older people demand foods to lower cholesterol and blood pressure. Finally, another relevant socio-demographic factor capable to influence the attitude of consumers towards FF pertains to the presence of young children in the household (Barrena and Sánchez, 2010; Maynard and Franklin, 2003). This factor may impact food choices because of its potential association with higher food risk aversion or higher quality consciousness, as exemplified for instance for fresh meat after the BSE crisis (e.g. Verbeke *et al.*, 2000).

3.2. Health Consciousness

Another important factor for the consumption of FF is the preservation of good health status (Urala 2005) and to what extent consumers perceive FF contribute to this aim. Many research has shown that FF appear to have benefitted from increased consumer awareness and interest in healthy lifestyles (ILC, UK 2010). Herath and colleagues (2008) suggest that consumers who demonstrate concern about a wide range of health issues are more receptive towards FF.

Particularly, European consumers consider food healthiness to be an important factor affecting their overall nutrition choices (Lappalainen *et al.*, 1998). Indeed healthiness is one of the most frequently mentioned motivations behind food choice in general (Saher *et al.*, 2004), as for FF. The main benefits mentioned by consumers are: general well-being, ease of following a healthy diet and prevention of diseases (Urala and Lähteenmäki, 2004, 2003; Bhaskaran and Hardley, 2002; Frewer *et al.*, 2003). The research by Urala and Lahteenmaki (2003), through laddering interviews, showed that consumers connect FF with: control over life and health, being a better person and feelings of well-being. In addition, use of FF may offer a new, less-demanding way of gaining an ethical reward through food choices, as consumers feel that they take care of themselves and make the right choice (Sirò *et al.*, 2008).

However, also in this case, there is a considerable body of research that demonstrates the existence of strong individual differences in health behavior (Armitage and Conner, 2000; Gilbert, 2000). Research by van Kleef, van Trijp and Luning (2005) proves that the relation between health condition of a consumer and the type of product's health claim affects the intention to buy the product. Similarly Lalor and colleagues (2011) demonstrated that positive attitudes towards FF seemed to rely on people's health (i.e. participants were more inclined to have a positive attitude if they were attempting to reverse a specific health issue). Also, Frewer, Scholderer and Lambert (2003) emphasize that consumer risk perceptions may have an important role in the acceptance of FF. Moreover perceived relevance increases the perceived benefit and makes products or concepts more appealing (Dean *et al.*, 2012). While surveys of Vassallo et al. (2009), de Jong, Ocké, Branderhorst, and Friele (2003), de Jong et al. (2004) showed that consumers' perceived state of health has only a limited influence on his or her choice of FF. Verbeke (2005) found that believing in the health effects of FF is the most crucial factor affecting consumer acceptance. Cox et al. (2004) found that the perceived efficacy accounted well for the intention to consume FF that were claimed to improve memory. Another important factor is the presence of specific health problems: according to Verbeke (2005) the existence of a family member with a particular health difficulty positively affects the acceptance of FF.

3.3. Sensory and Non-sensory Product Attributes

Several studies have shown that the attractiveness of FF does not depend only on their perceived healthiness, but it is influenced also by the product attributes as sensory quality (Urala and Lähteenmäki, 2007), as well as non-sensory factors, such as brand and price (Ares *et al.*, 2010; Ares and Gambaro, 2007), as any other conventional food product. According to these authors, consumers are not willing to negotiate those characteristics for eventual long-term health benefits.

With reference to sensory characteristics, taste is one of the most important factors that affect consumers' choice of FF (Verbeke, 2006; Urala, 2005) as well as the perception that FF could be less natural than conventional foods (Cox *et al.*, 2004; Frewer *et al.*, 2003). Numerous consumer studies have also pointed to the primary role of taste as a factor that directs consumers choice when selecting FF (Tuorila and Cardello, 2002; Gilbert, 2000; Poulsen, 1999; Childs and Poryzees, 1997). Previous research revealed that consumers in general are hardly willing to compromise on the taste of FF for possible health benefits. Verbeke (2006) indicates that consumers have become more convinced that good taste and healthiness are not necessarily to be traded-off against each other. However, Urala and Lahteenmaki (2004) indicate that some products may have such a strong health claim that consumers are still ready to compromise on taste.

On the other hand, several studies have pointed out that consumer perception of FF depends more on the perception of the nutritional qualities of the base product than on the functional ingredient.

Some scholars, outside Europe, demonstrated that carriers of functional ingredients had the largest relative importance in consumers valuation of FF (Hailu *et al.*, 2009; Cox *et al.*, 2008). Bech-Larsen and Grunert (2003) showed that the type of base product contributes to how much consumers perceive FF to be healthy. Van Kleef and colleagues (2005) add that potential buyers tend to trust more health claims when the basic carrier has a positive overall image, as well as a history in health claims (as yogurt and fruit juices). Conversely, foods that are perceived as unhealthy (e.g. mayonnaise) do not benefit from having an approved health claim (e.g. Miele *et al.*, 2010).

Another interesting result that emerges in literature is that functional ingredients which are familiar to consumers, tend to achieve higher rates of consumer acceptance (Siro *et al.*, 2008). Hence it is much easier to gain consumer acceptance for a product enriched with more familiar ingredients, such as vitamin C, calcium, Omega-3, than it is for unfamiliar ones, such as selenium (Bech-Larsen and Scholderer 2007; Menrad 2003).

Other researchers have focused their attention on the influence of non sensory factors. Among non-sensory attributes, brand and price have been identified by scholars as the most important underlying consumers' food choices. According to a study carried out by Ares et al. (2010) brand is a key factor influencing consumers' choice behaviour of functional yoghurt.

Price could influence consumer purchase intention in two different ways: lower purchasing intention due to a greater monetary sacrifice, or have a positive impact on purchase intention because of an increase perceived product quality. Indeed, according to several authors there is a group of consumers who are not affected by a price increase and are willing to pay premium price for FF (Bouge and Ryan, 2000; Poulsen, 1999). However, overall, consumers seem to be only willing to accept a limited price premium (Menrad, 2003).

Other non-sensory factors, beyond brand and price, that could influence consumers' attitudes toward FF are convenience and packaging. Specifically, Urala and Laatemaki (2003) identified convenience as an important factor in determining consumers choice of FF. Considering time constraints consumers would probably not be willing to compromise convenience for health related issues, so FF should be developed maintaining the convenience level of their conventional counterparts (Ares, 2011).

Also packaging might play an important role in influencing consumer attitudes towards FF. Since packaging is a source of product recognition and serves as an extrinsic quality cue, attracting consumers' attention and communicates important messages to the consumer (Moskowitz *et al.*, 2009). However, only few studies have analysed this particular attribute in the FF market (e.g. Ares *et al.*, 2010; Stein and Rodríguez-Cerezo, 2008).

3.4. Information and Health Claims

Benefits of FF may not be directly experienced by consumers, therefore producers must effectively communicate potential benefits to consumers. Consequently the type of information and the trust in it regarding the effect of a particular product on health represent crucial factors of FF success (Di Pasquale *et al.*, 2011; Urala, 2005). At the same time some studies report lack of information as a reason for not consuming, while others reveal an overload of information, especially if too scientific, tend to decrease overall acceptance (Verbeke, 2005). Bitzios, Fraser and Haddock-Fraser (2011) revealed that consumers tend to prefer FF products that carry a simple but clear health benefit.

Moreover, according to Del Giudice and Pascucci (2010) the acceptance of FF ingredients is influenced by the way consumers obtain their information and knowledge; however the intensity of information search depends on the level of personal involvement. Several studies show that consumer confidence in the information provided on FF may vary according to source. Annunziata and Vecchio (2010) reveal that Italian consumers had a high degree of confidence in information from doctors and public authorities, while a lower degree of confidence is accorded to manufacturers. Likewise Urala and Lähteenmäki (2003) show that Finnish consumers are very confident with health-related information coming from the authorities and quite confident with information reported by newspapers, retailers, and food producers. A Greek research (Pounis *et al.*, 2011) highlighted that an increase of iron nutrition knowledge was associated with 20% higher likelihood of consuming iron fortified foods more often. These results support the idea that information sourced from a trusted, credible, and recognizable agency may have a positive impact on the valuation and the likelihood of acceptance of FF. Several studies (Grunert *et al.*, 2009; Lähteenmäki *et al.*, 2010; van Trijp and van der Lans, 2007) have shown that previous exposure to FF seems to facilitate their acceptance, especially when claims have more detailed information. In particular, since health claims can play a role in guiding consumer purchasing decisions for FF literature has paid particular attention to this concern.

Nevertheless, in general, there seems to be relatively few consistent findings on consumers' responses to health claims (Lähteenmäki, 2012). There are several studies that have investigated consumer reactions towards different types of health claims (van Kleef *et al.*, 2005; van Trijp and van der Lans, 2007), while other studies have included measurement of the credibility of health claims (Labrecque *et al.*, 2006; Niva and Makela, 2007; van Kleef *et al.*, 2005) or the influence of health claims on willingness to pay for FF (Marette *et al.*, 2010, Mialon *et al.*, 2002).

Pothoulaki and Chryssochoidis (2009) report that consumers find disease risk reduction claims more appealing than other claims, particularly when the individual has experience of the disease concerned. Whereas Verbeke et al. (2009) found that health claims were more convincing than nutrition claims, and that disease risk reduction claims reduced credibility.

Other studies have revealed that consumers tend to trust health claims more when the basic carrier has a positive overall image (Siegrist *et al.*, 2008; Van Kleef *et al.*, 2005).

Urala and Lahteenmaki (2004) indicate that some products may have such a strong health claim that consumers are still ready to compromise on taste. Furthermore, while Marette et al. (2010) show that a significant and positive influence of the message linked to the cholesterol reduction exist on willingness to pay for FF, Mialon and colleagues (2002) attributed higher willingness to pay to the fact that most products in their study were already perceived as being high in fiber so additional information did not influence the acceptance ratings. Another study conducted by van Trijp and van der Lans (2007) on consumer acceptance of a yoghurt with various nutrition and health-related claims, suggest that consumer perception differs according to the benefit being claimed. Products with the added benefits of reducing the negative impact of stress or improving concentration had lower consumer appeal than products strengthening body's natural defense system. Furthermore, Van Kleef and colleagues (2005) explored carrier and health claim compatibility for 100 hypothetical products, not finding any significant interaction between health claim and carrier; revealing that consumer evaluation of health claims varies according to how much the claim is personally relevant to the consumer in addressing a disease they have experienced.

4. Main Differences among European Consumers

As already highlighted, demand for FF within the EU varies considerably from country to country, mainly due to food traditions and cultural heritage (Castellini *et al.*, 2002). These differences, along with differences in socio-economic features, can influence the greater or lesser propensity of consumers to new products concepts. Understanding this diversity of preferences and sensitivities that exist among consumers in the market is one of the greatest challenges in consumer and market research. Core differences between European consumers emphasize the need for public and private operators to know in depth (and take into account) these peculiarities when designing specific marketing strategies.

In this regards many scholars have focused on cross-country analysis of acceptance of FF. Most of such studies have demonstrated that cognitive, motivational and attitudinal determinants of consumer acceptance of FF vary considerably among countries. Moreover, also attitude towards health claims is known to be different in diverse countries partly because of different histories in use of health claims before the harmonization operated by EU legislation (Grunert *et al.*, 2011).

Frewer et al. (2003) presented a very informative review of various cross-cultural and demographic factors that could affect acceptance of FF. Some of the factors found to be important for acceptance of FF were: cross-cultural and intra-individual factors which may be related to nutritional knowledge; consumer perception of the technology used to produce the food (for example genetic modification); the degree to which sensory properties meet customer expectations; and the price of the food.

Other relevant studies point out that in general, interest of consumers towards FF in central and northern European states is higher than in Mediterranean countries (Van Trijp and van der Lans, 2007), this could also be related to a lower degree of penetration of such products in these latter markets and lower consumer awareness. For example, Niva (2000) as well as Makela and Niva (2002) and Niva and Makela (2007), indicated that the need for FF is increasingly questioned in Northern European countries, hence yielding the conclusion that consumer acceptance of FF cannot be taken for granted anymore. Bech-Larsen and Grunert (2003) reveal that attitudes toward FF were more positive in Finnish consumers compared to consumers in Denmark or USA. However, their outcomes indicated that although Finnish respondents were generally more positive towards FF than Americans, and even more compared to the Danish, the three samples showed little differences as regards the determinants of healthiness perception of FF.

Moreover, Krygier (2007) found that while 49% of consumers were familiar with the term 'functional food' in Belgium, the same was true only for 4% of Polish consumers.

Furthermore recent findings showed that Swedish consumers think FF compensate for an unhealthy lifestyle and should only be used when it is not possible to improve personal health through lifestyle changes (Landstrom *et al.*, 2009), whereas English consumers consider FF as an easy way to achieve healthy eating (Urala, 2005).

Other international studies have compared northern with Mediterranean European countries showing that knowledge and awareness of FF differed across national case studies. Stein and Rodríguez-Cerezo (2008) reveal that in Spain one third of the interviewees knew the term "functional food", in Germany and in Poland this share lowered to one fifth and only one out of ten respondents in the United Kingdom. Other relevant differences were found in the reasons for not buying FF. For instance, in Poland and in Spain the price of FF products was a much more important deterrent for purchasing than in the United Kingdom or in Germany. In addition the fear of side-effects is a more important reason among Polish respondents to reject FF than for British interviewees.

Other studies have focused their attention on country differences in consumers' perceptions of benefits relating to specific FF. Dean et al. (2010) in their study on functional cereal products demonstrate that British, Finns and Italians perceived cholesterol-lowering bread to be significantly more beneficial than the Germans. Furthermore, the British and the Italians perceived cholesterol-lowering pasta and biscuits as having more benefits than Finns and Germans.

Messina et al. (2008) in their research have investigated older people's perceptions of functional yoghurt across eight European countries (UK, Denmark, Germany, Poland, Portugal, Spain, Sweden and Italy). Findings demonstrate that for Italians, Spanish, Portuguese, Danish and Swedish the first principal axis in influencing older consumers towards functional yoghurt could be interpreted as what they defined novel-common axis, whilst in the UK, Germany and Poland other factors were more important. Recent work by Žeželj and colleagues (2012) in six Western Balkan countries demonstrated that healthiness was the first ranked attribute for FF and respondents also expected these products to be appealing to the senses.

Another aspect that has been investigated in literature regarding differences between various European countries is the perception of nutritional claims. Van Trijp and van Der Lans (2007) used a large-scale internet-based survey to investigate consumer perceptions of nutritional claims across different countries, revealing that consumers in different countries perceive nutritional health claims very differently. For example, the authors show that nutritional claims are relatively more difficult to understand in the UK than in Germany and Italy.

In addition, Stein and Rodríguez-Cerezo (2008) explained that for respondents in Germany and the United Kingdom the highest willingness to pay could be derived for the cancer prevention claims, in particular those with dietary fibers as ingredients. While in Spain the protection claim with lycopene seems to boost willingness to pay more than the cancer prevention claim.

5. Strategies for Development and Marketing of Functional Food

The objective of this review was not only to organize and review the large number of articles in the recent European FF literature, but also to critically examine what is nowadays clear accepted knowledge that is of value for the industry and policy makers.

Functional foods have been amply shown to represent a rapidly developing and particularly promising market segment. Even if European markets generally are less developed, compared to the US and the Japanese ones, FF already constitute a significant market in the EU with a large development potential.

Albeit several mid- and long-term developments in society, as well as socio-demographic trends, are in favor of FF raise, to the point that many authors tend to suppose that FF represents a sustainable category in the food market (Sirò *et al.*, 2008; Bech-Larsen and Scholderer, 2007; Jones and Jew, 2007; Van Kleef *et al.*, 2002), there are specific challenges in the development and marketing of such products.

To date the FF market is still characterized by a high rate of product failures. Despite the lack of exact data for this market in Europe it can be assumed that the product failure rate in this product segment most probably will continue to be elevated, due to the specific challenges in the development and marketing of FF (Sirò *et al.*, 2008; Bech-Larsen and Scholderer, 2007).

Analyses of past experiences, excluding functional dairy products, suggest that FF have developed in a very fragmented way in Europe so far. Most "functional" brands have been launched in a limited number of countries in recent years, moreover in many cases multinational food industry companies have introduced rather single products than fully developed umbrella brands in this market. This suggest that only products with a sufficient mass-market appeal managed to survive (Bech Larsen and Scholderer, 2007; Menrad, 2003).

In this context the future of FF market development is influenced by both consumers' degree of familiarity and acceptance as well opportunities originating in life sciences (Ares and Gambaro, 2007; Van Kleef *et al.*, 2002).

Almost all the studies that we have analyzed in this review reveal that consumer acceptance of the concept of FF together with a better understanding of its determinants are key factors for market orientation, development and market success. However, failure rates have shown that consumer acceptance is often neglected or at least far from being understood (Verbeke, 2005). As highlighted before, consumer acceptance of FF is a multifaceted phenomenon influenced by several factors which may also vary in different European countries.

Summarizing the findings of the most prominent studies reviewed it is possible to identify some key factors related to consumers acceptance of FF in Europe, representing at the present time also the major market challenges for FF manufacturers.

The first factor is the lack of familiarity of European consumers with FF. According to surveys in different European countries in many cases it is still difficult for consumers to distinguish between functional and conventional food products, because consumers often do not know the term "functional food" or similar phrasing (even if they show a rather high agreement to the concept). Clearly this factor denotes an increasing consumer confusion, maybe due to a lack of categorisation about the FF concept but also due to a fragmented product variety available on the market and to the great amount of general marketing and educational messages that are not coordinated with each other.

The second factor is connected to consumers' low awareness of health benefits of functional ingredients. The acceptance of a specific functional ingredient is linked to consumers' knowledge of the health effects of that specific ingredient. Many studies have showed that functional ingredients which are in the mind of consumers for a relatively long period of time achieve considerably higher rates of consumer acceptance than ingredients which are used for a short period of time. This is maybe due to the consumers' attitude to prefer naturalness in their foods and form negative associations in response to foods with highly specific functional components, particularly when communications use an excessively scientific wording.

As a consequence there is a strong need for specific information and communication activities, especially to foster development of new specific market segments (Biacs, 2007; Salminen, 2007; Wansink *et al.*, 2005; Menrad, 2003).

Consumers' perception and understanding of the health claims represent another key factor that influence acceptance of FF. As widely acknowledged, beyond providing consumer protection against unproven or untruthful statements, nutrition and health claims can help consumers to make better-informed food choices (Leathwood *et al.*, 2007; Williams and Ghosh, 2008). Simultaneously, nutrition and health claims can be considered as strong marketing incentives for food manufacturers since they allow product differentiation based on health-related positioning (Bech-Larsen and Scholderer, 2007; Cheftel, 2005).

However, as highlighted in the current review, previous studies led to the conclusion that consumers are skeptical of nutrition and health claims although they perceive those claims as potentially useful. Furthermore consumers do not clearly distinguish between different levels of health claims; tend to prefer succinct rather than complex claims; and consumer reactions depend upon the combination of carrier product, type of enrichment and health benefit claimed (Verbeke *et al.*, 2009).

In this regards it has been observed that products with highly specific functional or health claims, appealing only to small market niches, tended to fail particularly when communications used a negative or too scientific framing such as the prevention of specific diseases (Euromonitor, 2004). Conversely, Sirò et al. (2008) stated that sometimes products for which communications created a holistic health image (e.g. Danone's Actimel), often in a positive framing such as promotion of general well-being and the prolongation of youth, had superior market success.

Introduction of Regulation EC (No) 1924/2006[1] (European Commission, 2007) from January 2007, undoubtedly represents an important opportunity to design truthful and not misleading health claims, since its basis and its wording must be mandatory and fully consistent with scientific evidence. However, Bech-Larsen and Scholderer (2007) expressed skepticism towards the potential of the new legislation to enlarge the European market for FF due to the lack of correspondence between the new legislation, consumers' preferences and actual marketing experiences with this market segment.

[1] In Europe, the Health Claims regulation recognizes the work of the EC Concerted Actions FUFOSE (Functional Food Science in Europe) and PASSCLAIM (Process for the Scientific Support for Claims on Foods) as valuable projects to be taken into account when assessing health claims. Regulation EC (No) 1924/2006 allows basically two types of claims to be made on foodstuffs: nutrition claims and health claims. The latter can be divided into functional health claims and reduction of disease risk claims.

Given the previous considerations, the main challenge for FF in the next future will be to find/create a favorable identity. This could be done firstly by re-establishing FF perceived value by improving quality with regard to both taste and nutritional significance.

So it may be stated that to define the medium/long-term prospects of FF market there is an urgent need to increase investments in research and development to support innovation and increase the added value of these products. These innovations should try to answer as much as possible consumers' needs in terms of health requirements but also should take into account the central role of both sensory and non-sensory attributes (with particular reference to price, brand and packaging).

At the same time it is crucial to guarantee a proper and clear flow of information between businesses and consumers, enabling sound evaluation of the benefits that may result from the consumption of FF; and full consumer confidence in companies and bodies called to protect consumption. Information that considers the consumer's perspective can help FF manufacturers better connect with consumers and guide the latter ones towards informed and healthful food choices. Therefore, more clearly defined policies need to be developed for FF to avoid false health claims during the marketing process.

REFERENCES

AC Nielsen (2007). *What's hot around the globe—Insights on growth in alcoholic beverage categories*. New York: Author. [Date accessed: September 13, 2012]

Ares, G., Gimenez, A., & Deliza, R. (2010). Studying the influence of package shape and colour on consumer expectations of milk desserts using word association and conjoint analysis. *Food Quality and Preference*, 21, 361–367.

Armitage, C.J., & Conner, M. (2000). Social cognition models and health behaviour: A structured review. *Psychology and Health*, 15, 173–189.

Annunziata, A. & Vecchio, R. (2011). Functional foods development in the European market: A consumer perspective. *Journal of Functional Food*, 3, 223–228.

Anttolainen, M., Luoto, R., Uutela, A., Boice, J. D., Blot, W. T., McLaughlin, J. K., *et al.* (2001). Characteristics of users and nonusers of plant sterol margarine in Finland: an approach to study functional foods. *Journal of the American Dietetic Association*, 101, 1365–1368.

Ares, G., & Gambaro, A. (2007). Influence of gender, age and motives underlying food choice on perceived healthiness and willingness to try functional foods. *Appetite*, 49, 148–158.

Bhaskaran, S., & Hardley, F. (2002). Buyers beliefs, attitudes and behaviour: foods with therapeutic claims. *Journal of Consumer Marketing*, 19, 591–606.

Barrena, R., & Sánchez, M. (2010). The link between household structure and the level of abstraction in the purchase decision process: an analysis using a functional food. *Agribusiness*, 26 243–264.

Bech-Larsen, T., Grunert, K. G., & Poulsen, J. B. (2001). The acceptance of functional foods in Denmark, Finland and the United States. A study of consumers' conjoint evaluations of the qualities of functional food and perceptions of general health factors and cultural values. Working Paper No. 73. Aarhus, Denmark: MAPP.

Bech-Larsen, T., & Grunert, K. G. (2003). The perceived healthiness of functional foods— A conjoint study of Danish, Finnish and American consumers' perception of functional foods. *Appetite*, 40, 9–14.

Bech-Larsen, T., & Scholderer, J. (2007). Functional foods in Europe: Consumer research, market experiences and regulatory aspects. *Trends in Food Science & Technology*, 18, 231–234.

Biacs, P.A. (2007). Regulations and claims of functional foods. In Proceedings of the fourth International FFNet meeting on functional foods.

Bitzios, M., Fraser, I., & Haddock-Fraser, J., (2011). Functional ingredients and food choice: results from a dual-mode study employing means-end-chain analysis and a choice experiment. *Food Policy*, 36, 714–724.

Bleiel, J. (2010). Functional foods from the perspective of the consumer: How to make it a success? *International Dairy Journal*, 20, 303-306.

Bogue, J., & Ryan, M. (2000). *Market-oriented new product development: Functional foods and the Irish consumer*. Agribusiness Discussion Paper No. 27. Department of Food Economics, National University of Ireland, Cork.

Bonanno A. (2011). Functional foods as differentiated products: the Italian Yogurt Market, *European Review of Agricultural Economics*, 1–27.

Canavari, M., Castellini, A., Nocella, G., &. Pirazzoli, C. (2007). Functional foods in the European Union: Main issues and impact on the food industry. In Losso, J. N., Shahidi, F., and Bagchi, D., editors, *Anti-Angiogenic Functional and Medicinal Foods, Nutraceutical Science and Technology*, 6(Chapter 11): 251-274. CRC Press (Taylor & Francis Group), Boca Raton, FL, USA.

Cheftel, J.C. (2005). Food and nutrition labelling in the European Union. *Food Chemistry*, 93, 531–550.

Childs, N.M., & Poryzees, G.H. (1997). Foods that help prevent disease: Consumer attitudesand public policyimplications. *Journal of Consumer Marketing*, 14, 433–447.

Cox, D.N., Koster, A., & Russell, C.G. (2004). Predicting intentions to consume functional foods and supplements to offset memory loss using an adaptation of protection motivation theory. *Appetite*, 33, 55–64.

Cox, D.N., & Bastiaans, K. (2007). Understanding Australian consumers' perception of selenium and motivations to consume selenium-enriched foods. *Food Quality and Preference*, 18, 66–76.

Cox, D.N., Evans, G., & Lease, H.J. (2008). Australian consumers' preferences for conventional and novel sources of long chain omega-3 fatty acids: A conjoint study. *Food Quality and Preference*, 19, 306-314.

Dean, M., Lampila, P., Shepherd, R., Arvola, A., Saba, A., Vassallo, M., *et al.* (2012). Perceived relevance and foods with health-related claims. *Food Quality and Preference*, 24(1), 129–135.

De Jong, N., Ocké, M. C., Branderhorst, H. A. C., & Friele, R. (2003). Demographic and lifestyle characteristics of functional food consumers and dietary supplement users. *British Journal of Nutrition*, 89(2), 273–281.

De Jong, N., Verhaegen, H., Wolfs, M.C.J., Ocké, M.C, Klungel, O.H, & Leukens, H.G.M. (2007). Functional foods the case for closer evaluation. *British Medical Journal*, 334, 1037-1039.

Del Giudice, T., & Pascucci, S. (2010). The role of consumer acceptance in the food innovation process: Young consumer perception of functional foods in Italy. *International Journal on Food System Dynamics*, 2, 111-122.

Di Pasquale, J., Adinolfi, F., & Capitanio, F. (2011). Analysis of Consumer Attitudes and Consumers' Willingness to Pay for Functional Foods. *International Journal on Food System Dynamics*, 2, 181-193.

Doyon, M., & Labrecque, J. (2008). Functional foods: A conceptual definition. *British Food Journal*, 110(11), 1133-1149.

European Commission. (2007). Regulation (EC) No 1924/2006 of the European Parliament and of the Council of 20 December 2006 on nutrition and health claims made on foods. *Official Journal of the European Union*, L 12/3–L 12/18.

European Food Information Council (EUFIC) (2006). Available from: http://www.eufic.org/en/quickfacts/obesity.htm [Date accessed: September 9, 2012]

Euromonitor International (2009). *Functional foods: A world survey*. London.

European Food Information Council (EUFIC) (2006), Backgrounder –Functional foods, June 2006.

FAO (Food and Agriculture Organization of the United Nations) (2007). *Evaluation of health and nutritional properties of probiotics in foods*. [Date accessed: September 9, 2012]

Frewer, L., Scholderer, J., & Lambert, N. (2003). Consumer acceptance of functional foods: Issues for the future. *British Food Journal*, 105, 714–731.

Gilbert, L. (2000). The functional food trend: What's next and what Americans think about eggs. *Journal of the American College of Nutrition*, 19, 507S-512S.

Grunert, K.G., Scholderer, J., & Rogeaux, M., (2011). Determinants of consumer understanding of health claims. *Appetite,* 56, 269–277.

Grunert, K.G., Lähteenmäki, L., Boztug, Y., Martinsdottir, E., Ueland, O., Åström, A. et al. (2009). Perception of health claims among Nordic consumers. *Journal of Consumer Policy*, 32, 269–287.

Hailu, G., Boecker, A., Henson, S., & Cranfield, J. (2009). Consumer valuation of functional foods and nutraceuticals in Canada. A conjoint study using probiotics. *Appetite*, 52, 257-265.

Hellyer, N., Fraser, I.M., & Haddock-Fraser, J. (2012). Food Choice, Health Information and Functional Ingredients: An Experimental Auction Employing Bread, *Food Policy*, 37, 232–245.

Herath, D., Cranfield, J., & Henson, S. (2008). Who consumes functional foods and nutraceuticals in Canada? Results of cluster analysis of the 2006 survey of Canadians' demand for food products supporting health and wellness. *Appetite*, 51, 256-265.

Jaeger, S.R. (2006). Non-sensory factors in sensory science research. *Food Quality and Preference*, 17, 132–144.

Jago, D. (2009). Functional foods, market trends. Paper presented at the Functional Foods Symposium, Amsterdam, The Netherlands.

Jones, P. J., & Jew, S. (2007). Functional food development: Concept to reality. *Trends in Food Science & Technology,* 18, 387–390.

Kearney, J. (2010). Food consumption trends and drivers. *Phil. Trans. R. Soc. B* 365, 2793–2807.

Kotilainen, L., Rajalahti, R., Ragasa, C., & Pehu, E. (2006). Health enhancing foods: Opportunities for strengthening the sector in developing countries. Agriculture and Rural Development Discussion Paper 30.

Krutulyte, R., Scholderer, J., Hagemann, K. , Grunert, G.K., Elgaard, P., Nielsen, B. et al. (2008). Motivational factors for consuming omega-3 PUFAs: An exploratory study with Danish consumers. *Appetite*, 51, 137–147.

Krutulyte, R., Grunert, K.G., Scholderer, J., Lähteenmäki, L., Hagemann, K.S., Elgaard, P., Nielsen, B., & Graverholt, J.P. (2011). Perceived fit of different combinations of carriers and functional ingredients and its effect on purchase intention. *Food Quality and Preference* 22 (1), 11-17.

Krystallis, A., Maglaras, G., & Mamalis, S. (2008). Motivations and cognitive structures of consumers in their purchasing of functional foods. *Food Quality and Preference*, 19, 525-538.

Labrecque, J., Doyon, M., Bellavance, F., & Kolodinsky, J. (2006). Acceptance of functional foods. A comparison of French, American, and French Canadian consumers. *Canadian Journal of Agricultural Economics*, 54, 647–661.

Landstrom, E., Koivisto Hursti, U.K., & Magnusson, M. (2009). Functional foods compensate for an unhealthy lifestyle – some Swedish consumers' impressions and perceived need of functional foods. *Appetite*, 53, 34-43.

Lappalainen, R., Kearney, J., & Gibney, M. (1998). A pan European survey of consumer attitudes to food, nutrition, and health: An overview. *Food Quality and Preference*, 9, 467-478.

Lähteenmäki, L., (2012). Claiming health in food products. *Food Quality and Preference*, in press. http://dx.doi.org/10.1016/j.foodqual.2012.03.006

Lähteenmäki, L., Lampila, P., Grunert, K., Boztug, Y., & Ueland, Ø., (2010). Impact of health-related claims on the perception of other product attributes. *Food Policy*, 35, 230–239.

Leathwood, PD., Richardson, D.P., Sträter, P., Todd, P.M., & van Trijp, H.C. (2007). Consumer understanding of nutrition and health claims: sources of evidence. *British Journal of Nutrition*, 98(3), 474-484.

Luckow, T., & Delahunty, C. (2004). Consumer acceptance of orange juice containing functional ingredients. *Food Research International*, 37, 805–814.

Lyly, M., Roininen, K., Honkapaa , K., Poutanen, K., & Lahteenmaki, L. (2007). Factors influencing consumers' willingness to use beverages and ready-to-eat frozen soups containing oat b-glucan in Finland, France and Sweden. *Food Quality and Preference*, 18, 242–255.

Makinen-Aakula, M. (2006). Trends in functional foods dairy market. *Paper presented at the 3rd FFNet Meeting on Functional Foods*, Budapest, Hungary.

Marette, S., Roosen, J., Blanchemanche, S., & Feinblatt-Mélèze, E. (2010) Functional food, uncertainty and consumers' choices: A lab experiment with enriched yoghurts for lowering cholesterol. *Food Policy*, 35, 419–428.

Markovina, J., Cacic, J., Gajdoš, J., Kljusuric, D., & Kovacic, (2011). Young consumers' perception of functional foods in Croatia. *British Food Journal*, 113, 7-16.

Maynard, L.J., & Franklin, S.T. (2003). Functional foods as a value-added strategy: The commercial potential of cancer-fighting dairy products. *Review of Agricultural Economics*, 25, 316–331.

Menrad, K. (2003). Market and marketing of functional food in Europe. *Journal of Food Engineering*, 56, 181-188.

Messina F., Saba, A. Turrini, A., Raats, M., & Lumbers, M. (2008). Older people's perceptions towards conventional and functional yoghurts through the repertory grid method. A cross-country study. *British Food Journal* 8:790-804.

Miele, N.A., Di Monaco, R., Cavella, S., &. Masi, P. (2010). Effect of meal accompaniments on the acceptability of a walnut oil-enriched mayonnaise with and without a health claim. *Food Quality and Preference*, 21, 470–477.

Mintel (2011). Functional Food and Drink - UK - September 2011. [Date accessed: August 29, 2012]

Moskowitz, H., Reiner, M., Lawlor, J.B., & Deliza, R. (2009). *Packaging research in food product design and development.* Hoboken: Wiley–Blackwell.

Moskowitz, H., Beckley, J., & Minkus-McKenna, D. (2004). Use of conjoint analysis to assess web-based communications on functional foods. *Appetite*, 43, 85-92.

Niva, M. (2007). All foods affect health: Understandings of functional foods and healthy eating among health-oriented Finns. *Appetite*, 48, 384–393.

Niva, M., & Makela, J. (2007). Finns and functional foods: Sociodemographics, health efforts, notions of technology and the acceptability of health-promoting foods. *International Journal of Consumer Studies*, 31, 34-45.

Organic Monitor, (2009). *Global organic market. Time for organic plus strategies.* www.organicmonitor.com/r2905.htm [Date accessed: September 17, 2012]

Pothoulaki, M., & Chryssochoidis, G. (2009). Health claims: consumer's matters. *Journal of Functional Foods*, 1 (2), 222-228.

Poulsen, J. B. (1999). Danish consumers' attitudes towards functional foods. *Working Paper* No. 62. Aarhus, Denmark: MAPP.

Pounis, G.D., Makri, S., Gougias, L., Makris, H., Papakonstantinou, M., Panagiotakos, D.B., & Kapsokefalou, M. (2011). Consumer perception and use of iron fortified foods is associated with their knowledge and understanding of nutritional issues. *Food Quality and Preference*, 22, 683–688.

Roberfroid, M.B. (2000). An European consensus of scientific concepts of functional foods. *Nutrition*, 16, 689–691.

Saher, M., Arvola, A., Lindeman, M., & Lahteenmaki, L. (2004). Impressions of functional food consumers. *Appetite*, 42, 79–89.

Salminen, S. (2007). Health claim opportunities within probiotics and prebiotics. In Proceedings of the fourth international FFNet meeting on functional foods.

Siegrist, M., Sampfli, N., & Kastenholz, H. (2008). Consumers' willingness to buy functional foods. The influence of carrier, benefit and trust. *Appetite*, 51, 526–529.

Siro, I., Kapolna, E., Kapolna, B., & Lugasi, A. (2008). Functional food. Product development, marketing and consumer acceptance – a review. *Appetite,* 51, 456-467.

Sparke, K., & Menrad, K. (2009). Cross-European and Functional Food-Related Consumer Segmentation for New Product Development. *Journal of Food Products Marketing,* 15 (3), 213-230.

Stein, A.J., & Rodriguez-Cerezo, E. (2008). Functional food in the European Union. European Commission JRC Scientific and Technical Reports EUR 23380 EN.

Stewart-Knox, B. J., Vaz De Almeida, M. D., Parr, H., Pinhao, S., Bunting, B., & Gibney, M. (2007). Consumer uptake of functional foods in Europe. International developments in science & health claims, *ILSI international symposium on functional foods in Europe.*

Szakály, Z., Szente, V., Kövér, G., Polereczki, Z., & Szigeti, O. (2011). The influence of lifestyle on health behavior and preference for functional foods. *Appetite*, 58, 406–413.

Tuorila, H., & Cardello, A.V. (2002). Consumer responses to an off-flavor in juice in the presence of specific health claims. *Food Quality and Preference*, 13, 561-569.

Urala, N. (2005). *Functional foods in Finland: Consumers' views, attitudes and willingness to use*. Finland: VTT Publications.

Urala, N., & Lähteenmäki, L. (2003). Reasons behind consumer's functional food choices. *Nutrition and Food Science*, 33 (4), 148-158.

Urala, N., & Lahteenmäki, L. (2007). Consumers' changing attitudes towards functional foods. *Food Quality and Preference,* 18, 1-12.

Van Kleef, E., Van Trijp, H.C.M., Luning, P., & Jongen, W.M.F. (2002). Consumer oriented functional food development: How well do functional disciplines reflect the 'voice of the consumer'? *Trends in Food Science & Technology*, 13, 93–101.

Van Kleef, E., Van Trijp, H.C. M., & Luning, P. (2005). Functional foods: Health claim food product compatibility and the impact of health claim framing on consumer evaluation. *Appetite,* 44, 299-308.

van Trijp, H.C.M., & van der Lans, I.A. (2007). Consumer perceptions of nutrition and health claims. *Appetite*, 48, 305-324.

Vassallo, M., Saba, A., Arvola, A., Dean, M., Messina, F., Winkelmann, M., et al. (2009). Willingness to use functional breads. Applying the Health Belief Model across four European countries. *Appetite*, 52, 452-460.

Verbeke, W. (2005). Consumer acceptance of functional foods: Sociodemographic, cognitive and attitudinal determinants. *Food Quality and Preference,* 16, 45-57.

Verbeke, W. (2006). Functional foods: Consumer willingness to compromise on taste for health? *Food Quality and Preference,* 17, 126-131.

Verbeke, W.,Ward, R. W., & Viaene, J. (2000). Probit analysis of fresh meat consumption in Belgium: exploring BSE and television communication impact. *Agribusiness*, 16, 215–234.

Verbeke, W., Scholderer, J., & Lähteenmäki. L. (2009). Consumer appeal of nutrition and health claims in three existing product concepts. *Appetite*, 52, 684-692.

Wansink, B., Westgren, R.E., & Cheney, M.M. (2005). Hierarchy of nutritional knowledge that relates to the consumption of a functional food. *Nutrition,* 21, 264-268.

Williams, P., & Ghosh, D. (2008). Health claims and functional foods. *Nutrition & Dietetics*, 65, S89–S93.

In: Functional Foods
Editors: Aron Robinson and Dominick Emerson
ISBN: 978-1-62417-435-3

Chapter 5

FERMENTATION OF TOMATO JUICE WITH THE PROBIOTIC YEAST *SACCHAROMYCES CEREVISIAE BOULARDII*

Florinda Fratianni, Federica Cardinale, Ida Russo, Carmine Iuliano, Anna Carmela Cucciniello, Mena Maione, Antonio d'Acierno and Filomena Nazzaro*

Istituto di Scienze dell'Alimentazione, ISA-CNR, Avellino, Italy

ABSTRACT

A new functional beverage based on tomato juice fermented with the probiotic yeast *Saccharomyces cerevisiae boulardii* was formulated. Viability of the yeast, assayed after 24 h of incubation in the tomato juice and over 56 days of storage of the fermented product at 4°C, was comparable to that obtained by culturing the yeast in potato dextrose broth, used as a control. Therefore, the different culturing media did not negatively affect the yeast resistance to the *in vitro* passage through acidic and pancreatic environment. Some biochemical parameters of the fermented juice, polyphenol and lycopene content, as well as its DPPH free radical scavenging capability, were evaluated during storage and under *in vitro*-simulated gastrointestinal conditions. Fermentation of the juice with *S. boulardii* caused only a slight decrease of total polyphenols (0.442 μmol/μl *versus* 0.474 μmol/μl, respectively) and lycopene (13.38 μg/ml *versus* 16.76 μg/ml, respectively), compared to the raw juice. On the other hand, after passage through *in vitro* double gastric+ pancreatic conditions, the amount of such bio-components was constant during storage until 28 days, decreasing only after 56 days. Probably, such behaviour affected the slight loss of DPPH radical scavenging activity of the fermented juice with respect to the fresh product, and a decrease of 14% with respect to the initial value (EC_{50}= 38.54 μl) was observed after 56 days of storage (EC_{50}= 44.36 μl), although, after the double *in vitro* gastric+pancreatic passage, the amount of fermented juice request to inhibit the DPPH activity of 50% increased three times. The developed product might represent

* E-mail: mena@isa.cnr.it.

another example of an alternative for delivering probiotics, especially for individuals suffering from lactose intolerance to dairy products.

State of Art

Tomato is one of major vegetables widely consumed around the world. Italy, with about 5.9 million tons of tomato produced/year is one of the most important producers in the world [1]. The domestic production of tomato is addressed, for 14%, to the market of fresh produce; on the other hand, 86% of the Italian tomato production is processed [2]. In the world, tomatoes are processed for a wide range of products such as canned and sun-dried tomatoes, ketchups, pastes, purees, salads, sauces, soups, and juice products, supplying significant sources of vitamins and minerals to the consumers. The health benefits of fresh and processed tomatoes are attributed to the abundance of antioxidant components [3-5], which play an essential role as "health-promoting" agents in the diet. The most important biocomponent of tomato is lycopene, a carotenoid of which tomato is the principal source, giving to the fruit the characteristic red color and which, for its molecular structure and hydrophobic nature, is an effective antioxidant (Figure 1). More than 80% of dietary lycopene consumed in the diet come from a wide variety of tomato products [6].

Many processed tomato-based products provide more lycopene than the fresh fruit, where the molecule is present in a "trans" form; following the industrial process, lycopene can modify its spatial conformation, forming "cis" isomers, that appear to be more bioavailable for the body [7]. Among tomato products, juices are well recognized as healthy beverages and, with tomato paste and sauces, represent the main contributors of dietary lycopene intake [8]. There are extensive efforts to enhance the functionality of tomato juice by introducing other value-added components in the product. One of the interesting methods is represented by the so-called "probiotication", using microorganisms with probiotic properties and capable of having healthy effects [9]. The health effects attributed to the probiotics are numerous and well documented: contrast to diarrhea associated with antibiotics, rotavirus, chemotherapy, and traveller's diarrhea; stimulation of humoral and cellular immunity; decrease in unfavorable metabolites, such as ammonium and pro-cancerogenic enzymes in the colon. Furthemore, they act balancing positively the microbioma, hindering the action of pathogens (e.g. *Helicobacter pylori*), reduce allergic symptoms and irritable bowel syndrome; they have beneficial effects on mineral metabolism, particularly bone density and stability, and in cancer prevention and several strains are capable of reducing cholesterol and triacylglycerol plasma concentrations [10].

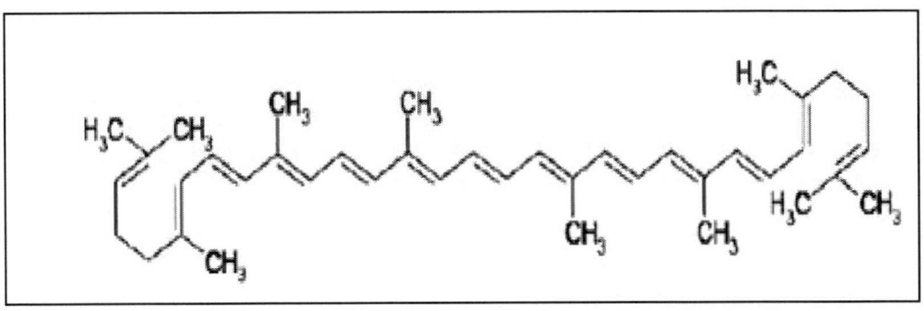

Figure 1. Structure of lycopene.

Supplements of probiotics to food may provide several health benefits including reduction in the level of serum cholesterol, improvement of gastrointestinal function, enhancement of the immune system, effectiveness against colon pathogens, reduction in risk of colon cancer [11,12] and, more recently, they were proven to give an important aid in the pathogenesis of diabetes and other metabolic diseases [13]. Probiotics must be consumed regularly at a sufficiently high number of viable and highly functional cells, and a daily minimum of 10^8 cells was proposed to ensure probiotic effects on consumers' health [9]. It has been suggested that fruit or vegetable juice could serve as a good medium for culturing probiotics [14-17]. Furthermore, they do not contain any dairy allergens that might prevent usage by certain segments of the population. *Lactobacillus* and *Bifidobacterium* strains are the most studied as probiotic agents because they are usual occupants of the intestinal tracts of humans and other vertebrates, and are frequently used to produce fermented products. So far, the active use of yeasts as dietary adjuncts for humans has been limited, in spite of the presence of yeasts, as an integral part of the microflora of many dairy-related products [18]. This might indicate that the potential of yeasts for incorporation into functional products as probiotic agents has been ignored or limited. Yeasts are microorganisms of huge economical attention, and play an essential role in the traditional as well as in modern biotechnology. During the last decades, *Saccharomyces cerevisiae boulardii* has been considered as a probiotic for human use and animal production. *S. boulardii* is a thermophilic non-pathogenic yeast, resistant to the gastric acidity and proteolysis [19]; in the gastrointestinal tract, it reaches a high level in a very short time and persists in viable forms. This yeast is generally administered, mainly in western Europe, for the prevention and treatment of a variety of diarrheal diseases, such as acute gastroenteritis in adults and children, antibiotic-associated diarrhea, diarrhea in tube-fed patients, and chronic diarrhea in HIV-infected patient. Clinical and experimental studies proved that oral treatment with *S. boulardii* can have beneficial effects in preventing the occurrence of complications linked to changes in the normal gut flora [20,21]. Several specific antagonistic interactions have been reported between culture yeasts like *S. boulardii* and some enteric pathogens, such as the enteropathogenic *Esherichia coli*, *Shigella* and *Salmonella* [19]. The use of probiotics yeasts such as *S. boulardii* in the formulation of functional fruity or vegetal probiotic foods is still underexploited; therefore, the effectiveness of a new functional tomato juice fermented with *S. boulardii* was evaluated, monitoring some biochemical aspects of the products and the viability of the probiotic yeast after passage through simulated gastro-intestinal conditions and during the storage of the product for eight weeks at 4°C.

EXPERIMENTAL

Saccharomyces cerevisiae boulardii was purchased in dried form in a local pharmacy in Napoli, Italy. Cells were reactivated in potato dextrose broth (Oxoid, Milano, Italy) at 37°C for 18 h. Pellets were washed in sterile physiological solution (NaCl 8.5 g/l) and resuspended in the same solution. A commercial pasteurized product, containing 100% tomato juice was used as the growth medium. Fermentation experiments were conducted in test tubes, each of them containing 30 ml of tomato juice. All samples were inoculated with the 18 h cultures (final concentration $>10^7$). After 24 hours of fermentation at 37°C, the fermented samples were stored at 4°C for 8 weeks. Samples were taken at 7, 14, 28 and 56 days, and viability of the culture in the fermented tomato juice was determined and expressed as $\log_{10}$ of colony-forming units (cfu)/ml of juice. Resistance to simulated gastric and intestinal juices was carried out using artificial gastric juice (potato dextrose broth, plus 3 g/l pepsin, at a final pH adjusted to 2.0) and artificial intestinal juice (potato dextrose broth plus 1 g/l pancreatin and 4.5 g/l bile salts), previously filter-sterilized (0.22 μm, Millipore SpA, Milano, Italy). The strain was treated using the protocol of De Giulio et al. [22], adopting an incubation in artificial gastric juice for 180 min at 37°C, and in pancreatic juice for 60 min at 37°C. Cell viability (cfu/ml) was evaluated by culturing on potato dextrose agar plates (37°C, 24 h) before and after incubation in the double passage gastric+pancreatic juices. Serial dilutions were prepared in sterile physiological solution before plating. Plates were incubated at 37° C for 24 h. *S. boulardii* grown in potato dextrose broth was used as control and treated in the same conditions. For biochemical analysis, tomato juice was centrifuged at 11,600 × *g* for 10min (Biofuge, Beckman, Los Angeles, CA, USA). The supernatant was used for biochemical analyses.

The content of total polyphenols of the product was spectrophotometrically evaluated (Cary 50 Uv/Vis, Varian-Agilent Italia, Cernusco sul Naviglio, Italy) at λ =760 nm, following the method described by Singleton and Rossi [23] with Folin-Ciocalteau reagent, using quercetin as standard. The results were expressed as μmol quercetin equivalent/μl sample. Antioxidant activity was measured with respect to the radical scavenging ability of the antioxidants present in the sample using the stable radical 2,2-diphenyl-1-picrylhydrazyl (DPPH) [24]. The analysis was performed by adding sample to a methanol solution (1:20 v/v) of DPPH (153 mM). The decrease in absorbance was determined with a UV-visible spectrophotometer (Cary, Varian, USA). The absorbance of DPPH radical without an antioxidant was used as a control. All determinations were in triplicate. The activity was calculated as EC_{50} defined as the amount of sample (μl) capable to inhibit 50% the activity of 1 ml DPPH activity after incubation at 60 minutes. Lycopene was extracted in hexane:methanol:aceton (2:1:1) plus 2.5% BHT (Butylhydroxytoluene) [25]. The absorbance was spectrophotometrically read at λ=450 nm and 503 nm (Cary 50 Uv/Vis , Varian-Agilent Italia, Cernusco sul Naviglio, Italy). The amount of lycopene (μg/ml) was calculated by the formula A_{450} x(ε)– A_{503} x (ε), with ε (450)= 3.956, and ε (503)= 0.806. Three replicates were carried out for each analysis. Statistical significance was performed as described in De Giulio et al. [22] and set at $P < 0.05$.

RESULTS

Microbial Analysis

Saccharomyces cervisiae boulardii was capable of using tomato juice as a growth medium, reaching 7.265 ± 0.023 log cfu/ml after 24 hours of incubation (Figure 2). Such value was similar to that obtained when the strain was grown in potato dextrose broth, demonstrating that tomato juice might be utilized by the yeast for its cell synthesis without nutrient supplementation or pH adjustment. The resulting product contained a number of cells aligned with the necessary doses of probiotics required to improve human health.

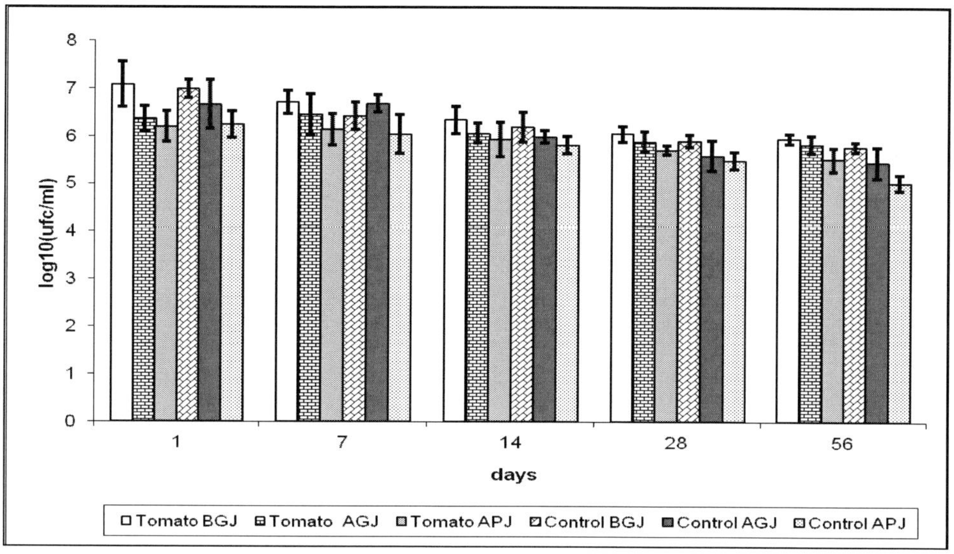

Figure 2. Viability (expressed as $\log_{10}$ cfu/ml) of *S.cerevisiae boulardii* grown in tomato juice or in potato dextrose broth (used as control), before gastric (BGJ), after gastric (AGJ) and after pancreatic (APJ) passage, monitored after 24 h, and until 56 days of storage at 4°C.

Therefore, suitability of tomato juice as an excellent medium for different probiotics has been extensively ascertained. Koh et al. [26], used the juice to formulate a new beverage containing bifidobacteria; Di Cagno et al. [27] assayed the potentialities of autochthonous lactic acid bacteria starters to improve the health and sensory properties of the tomato juice; some lactobacilli were used to ferment tomato juice by Yoon et al. [28] and Tsen et al. [29], which evaluated the effectiveness of the process applied by monitoring some microbial and chemical aspects of the fermented product for 4 weeks.

Data reported in Figure 2 also shows the effect of passage of the yeast through simulated gastric and pancreatic conditions. As in the control, a decrease of 1 logarithmic unit of cfu/ml was recorded after the double passage of *S. boulardii* grown in tomato juice through gastric+pancreatic juices, indicating that the different culturing media used in our experimentation did not negatively affect the yeast resistance to the *in vitro* stress conditions compared to the control. Viability of *S.boulardii* grown in tomato juice was maintained during the time of storage at 4°C, 56 days, taken into consideration; in light of an excellent behavior of the strain after 56 days (which gave still 7.197± 0.021 $\log_{10}$ cfu/ml), just a small decrease of its viability was observed after the simulation of the in vitro gastrointestinal stress (7.008 $\log_{10}$ cfu/ml). Such values were higher than those exhibited by the control (6.251 $\log_{10}$ cfu/ml and 5.852 $\log_{10}$ cfu/ml, respectively), confirming not only that tomato juice can be used to grow the probiotic yeast, but also that it might be more suitable for its growth and physiological functions; therefore, the capability of vegetable juices to more effectively protect microbial activity, as a whole, has been ascertained in the case of carrot juice that, when used as a growth medium for two strains of lactobacilli, was more capable to protect them against the simulated gastrointestinal stress than the conventional medium [14]; indeed, the concentration of the yeast cells, over 56 days of storage and after the simulated gastrointestinal stress, was still enough to answer to requirements to achieve beneficial effects.

Biochemical Analyses

Raw fruit or vegetable juices are usually strongly acidic solutions, containing from 10 to 25% soluble sugars. Generally, such situations might be considered highly suitable for the growth of yeasts and molds which naturally are contained in the raw fruit or vegetable juice, giving rise from the vegetable surface. As parts of the well known yeast-based fermented products, such as wine and beer, there are some fermented drinks and beverages made from fruit and vegetables, produced in Africa, Asia and Latin America, based on fermentation by yeasts of banana, cashew apples and other fruit juices, which maintain their biochemical characteristics [30]. In our experiment, tomato juice was used as a growth medium for a probiotic yeast strain, to evaluate the potential suitability of such matrix to constitute the basis of a new functional fermented juice, which, further to supply the body with probiotics, might retain its healthy peculiarities in terms of polyhenol and lycopene content, as well as the antioxidant activity. In the Chart 1, the polyhenol content exhibited by the fermented juice after 24 hours and during storage at 4°C until 8 weeks is shown. The uninoculated juice showed a content of polyphenols of about 0.474 μmol/μl . Such value did not decrease after 24 hours of fermentation with *S. boulardii*, giving a Δ= 0.028 μmol/μl; on the other hand, the values were constant after 56 days of storage at 4°C. A decrease of about 25%, respect to the situation observed before treatment with simulated gastrointestinal stress, was observed only at the end of the period considered, when the value was reduced from 0.463 μmol/μl before treatment with gastric juice to 0.358 μmol/μl, after passage with the pancreatic one . Such results are in agreement with Bermudez-Soto et al [31], which reported the sensitivity of dietary polyphenols to the alkaline conditions of the intestine, but are in contrast with Wootton-Beard et al [32], which showed that the polyphenol content was higher after digestive processes if compared to the levels prior of digestion. Probably, the lower amount of polyphenols observed in our experimentation might depend on the fermentation carried out by *S. boulardii* which, growing in tomato juice, could cause some chemical modifications, as demonstrated in other beverages by Rekha and Vijayalakshmi [33], and perhaps lead to a loss of its initial amount of polyphenols. In any case, although our results show that the concentration of phenolic compounds amount of polyphenol under the conditions of the small intestine is lower than in the fresh juice, it has to be taken into consideration that tomato juice remains, also after the digestive treatment, an important source of phenolic compounds with proven antioxidant activities. The antioxidant power of the tomato juice was measured through its capability to inhibit the activity of stable free radical DPPH and calculated in terms of EC_{50}, the volume (in μl) need to cut the radical activity of 50%.

Chart 1. Content of total polyphenols in the fermented tomato juice monitored after 24 h before gastric (BG) and after gastric+pancreatic (AGP) passages until 56 days of storage at 4°C. The data is expressed as μmol of quercetin equivalent/μL of juice

	T=0	24 h	7 days	14 days	28 days	56 days
BG	0.474 (±0.021)	0.442 (±0.015)	0.464 (±0.0105)	0.441 (±0.025)	0.426 (±0.009)	0.463 (±0.023)
AGP			0.457 (±0.0104)	0.456 (±0.009)	0.453 (±0.038)	0.358 (±0.014)

Chart 2. The DPPH radical scavenging activity (EC_{50}) of the fermented tomato juice monitored after 24 h before gastric (BG) passage and before gastric and after gastric+pancreatic (AGP) passage until 56 days of storage at 4°C

	0	24h	7 days	14 days	28 days	56 days
BG	33.34 (±1.24)	38.54 (±2.57)	34.87 (± .16)	46.06 (± 3.03)	47.98 (±3.45)	44.36 (±3.17)
AGP			113.36 (±8.95)	102.54 (±9.87)	103.56 (± 10.09)	175.54 (±15.42)

The results are shown in Chart 2. In fresh product, the EC_{50} was of about 33.34 µl; fermentation did not cause an evident loss of its antioxidant power (EC_{50}= 38.54 µl).

During 8 weeks of storage of the fermented product, its antioxidant activity decreased slowly, with a value inferior only of 14% respect to the initial value, after 56 days. After *the in vitro* digestion, the volume of fermented juice requested to inhibit the DPPH activity of 50% increased more than three times after 7 days of storage and four times at the end of the time considered. However, such behavior, in our opinion, was not determined by the presence of *S. boulardii*, but by probable intrinsic chemical modifications taking place within the product during storage. Probably, the double passage through simulated gastric and pancreatic environments might have induced a structural transformation of the product. The pH of a substance is known to affect racemisation of molecules, possibly creating two chiral enantiomers with different reactivity in the respective reagents. This might modify their biological reactivity, so that the antioxidants could be more reactive early in the digestive process, in particular, at the acidic pH of the gastric phase, and, conversely, less reactive at pH 7.4 in the duodenal phase, as racemisation can increase with pH in other compounds [34].

Therefore, the negative effect of digestion on the antioxidant activity of vegetal products is well reported in literature: after an *in vitro* digestive process, the bioavailability of the polyphenol fraction of olive oil decreases in a dramatic manner from 90% to 37%, with a negative effect on its antioxidant activity [35]. Such behavior, even though less evident, was observed in a red fruit juice enriched with pycnogenol [36], confirming that the great variability of polyphenols and the effect of digestion on them, with the subsequent variation of their intrinsic properties do not admit a unique answer and explanation. The content of lycopene decreased from the initial 19.65 µg/ml of the uninoculated juice to 16.76 µg/ml after fermentation, confirming that *S.boulardii* did not cause a marked adverse effect on lycopene content in tomato juice. (chart 3), neither negatively affected its nutritional value.

After 7 days of storage, the value decreased another 6% in respect to the fermentation, but it was constant until 4 weeks, diminishing just 2% after 56 days of storage at 4°C. Such a trend was observed also after treatment with gastrointestinal juices. Thus, tomato juice can be considered a good medium for the growth of different probiotics, also different from lactic acid bacteria, which do not negatively affect the health benefits of lycopene, that can be absorbed in adequate levels at the intestinal level, contributing-due to its unique structural and chemical features-to specific and biological properties in the protection of body against different kinds of cancer and cardiovascular diseases [7]. From the results of this study, it is concluded that *S. boulardii* could be used as probiotic culture for production of a new tomato juice-based functional beverage, for vegetarians or consumers allergic to lactose present in probiotic dairy products.

Chart 3. Content of lycopene (expressed as μg/ml of sample) present in the fermented tomato juice, monitored after 24 h before gastric (BG) passage and before gastric and after gastric+pancreatic (AGP) passage until 56 days of storage at 4°C

	0	24h	7 days	14 days	28 days	56 days
BG	19.65 (±3.45)	16.76 (±2.76)	13.38 (±1.95)	14.29 (±2.01)	13.52 (± 1.76)	12.92 (± 1.42)
AGP			13.11 (± 1.95)	14.92 (± 2.01)	13.67 (± 1.87)	10.59 (± 1.02)

REFERENCES

[1] World Processing Tomato Council, http://www.wptc.to/tomato-health-wptc.aspx.

[2] ISTAT – Informatic system on agriculture and zootecnics, 2009, www.istat.it.

[3] Giovannucci, E. (1999). Tomatoes, tomato-based products, lycopene, and cancer: review of the epidemiologic literature. *J. Natl. Cancer Inst.* 1990, 91,317–331.

[4] Rodriguez-Amaya, D.B., Tavares, C.A. Importance of cis-isomer separation in determining provitamin A in tomato and tomato products. *Food Chem.*1992,45,297-302.

[5] Hanson, P.M., Ledesma, D., Tsou, S.C.S., Lee, T.C., Yang, R., Wu, J., Chen, J. Variation of antioxidant activity and antioxidants in tomato. *J. Am. Soc. Hort. Sci.* 2004, 129,704–11.

[6] Willcox, J.K., Catignani, G.,L., Lazarus, S. Tomatoes and cardiovascular health. *Crit. Rev. Food Sci. Nutr.* 2003,43,1–18.

[7] Clinton, S.K. Lycopene: Chemistry, Biology, and Implications for Human Health and Disease. *Nutr. Rev.* 1998, 56, 35-51.

[8] Minorsky, P.V. Lycopene and the prevention of prostate cancer: the love apple lives up to its name. *Plant Physiol.* 2002, 130, 1077-1088.

[9] Guidelines for the evaluation of probiotics in food: Report of a joint FAO/WHO working group on drafting guidelines for the evaluation of probiotics in food. London: FAO/WHO 2002. Available in: ftp://ftp.fao.org/es/esn/food/wgreport2.pdf.

[10] Saarela, M., Lähteenäki, L., Crittenden, R., Salminen, S., Mattila- Sandholm, T. Gut bacteria and health foods - the European perspective. *Int. J. Food Microbiol.* 2002, 78, 99-117.

[11] Berner, L., O'Donnell, J. Functional foods and health claims legislation: Applications to dairy foods. *Int. Dairy J.* 1998, 8, 355-362.

[12] Rafter, J. Probiotics and colon cancer. *Best Prac. Res. Cli. Gastroentrol.* 2003,17, 849-859.

[13] Sanz, Y., Santacruz, A., Gauffin, P. Gut microbiota in obesity and metabolic disorders. *Proc. Nutr.Soc.* 2010, 69, 434-441.

[14] Fratianni, F., Coppola, R., Sada, A., Mendiola, J. A., Ibáñez, E., Nazzaro, F. A novel functional probiotic product containing phenolics and anthocyanins. *Int. J. Prob. Preb.* 2010. 5, 85-90.

[15] Nazzaro, F., Fratianni, F., Sada, A., Orlando, P. Synbiotic potential of carrot juice supplemented with Lactobacilli and inulin or fructooligosaccharides. *J. Sci. Food Agric.* 2008, 88, 2271-2276.

[16] Luckow, T., Delahunty, C. Which juice is healthier? A consumer study of probiotic non-dairy juice drinks. *Food Qual. Prefer.*2004,15,751–759.

[17] Granato, D., Branco, G.F., Nazzaro, F., Cruz, A.G., Faria, J.A.F. Functional foods and non-dairy probiotic food development: trends, concepts, and products. *Compr. Rev. Food Sci. Food Saf.* 2010, 9, 292-302.

[18] Fleet, G. H. Yeasts in dairy products. *J. Appl. Bacteriol.* 1990,68,199–211.

[19] Gedek, B.R. Regulierung der darmflora Uber die. *Nahrung Z. Hyg.* 1991, 191, 277–301.

[20] Czerucka, D., Piche, T., Rampal, P. Review article: yeast as probiotics – *Saccharomyces boulardii. Aliment. Pharmacol. Ther.* 2007, 26,767–778.

[21] Mcfarland, L. V., Bernasconi, P. *Saccharomyces boulardii*: A Review of an Innovative Biotherapeutic Agent. *Microb. Ecol. Health Dis.* 1993, 6, 157-171.

[22] De Giulio, B., Orlando, P., Barba, G., Coppola, R., De Rosa, M., Sada, A., De Prisco, P.P., Nazzaro, F. Use of alginate and cryo-protective sugars to improve the viability of lactic acid bacteria after freezing and freeze-drying. *W. J. Micr. Biotec.* 2005, 21, 739-746.

[23] Singleton, S.L., Rossi J.A. Colorimetry of total phenolics with phosphomolybdic-phosphotungstic acid reagents. *Am. J. Enol. Vitic.* 1965, 16, 144–158.

[24] Brand-Williams, W., Cuvelier, M.E., Berset, C. Use of a free radical method to evaluate antioxidant activity. *LWT - Food Sci. Technol.* 1995, 28, 25–30.

[25] Sharma, S.K., Le Maguer, M. Kinetics of lycopene degradation in tomato pulp solids under different processing and storage conditions. *Food Res. Int.* 1996, 29, 309–315.

[26] Tsen, J.H, Lin, Y.P., Huang, H.Y., King, V.A. Studies on the fermentation of tomato juice by using k-carrageenan immobilized *Lactobacillus acidophilus. J. Food Process. Preserv.* 2008, 32, 178–89.

[27] Di Cagno, R., Surico, R.F., Paradiso, A., Angelis, M.D., Salmon, J.C., Buchin, S., Gara, L.D., Gobbetti, M. Effect of autochthonous lactic acid bacteria starters on health-promoting and sensory properties of tomato juices. *Int. J. Food Microbiol.* 2009, 128, 473–83.

[28] Yoon, K.Y., Woodams, E.E., Hang, Y.D. Probiotication of tomato juice by lactic acid bacteria. *J. Microbiol.* 2004, 42, 315–318.

[29] Koh, J.H., Kim,Y., Jun-Hyun Oh, J.H. Chemical characterization of tomato juice fermented with bifidobacteria. *J. Food Sci.* 2010, 75, C428-C432.

[30] Battcock, M., Azam Ali, S. Fermented fruits and vegetables. A global perspective. *FAO Agricultural Services Bulletin,* 1998,134, pp.0-99. Rome, Italy.

[31] Bermúdez-Soto, M.J., Tomás-Barberán, F.A., García-Conesa, M.T. Stability of polyphenols in chokeberry (*Aronia melanocarpa*) subjected to *in vitro* gastric and pancreatic digestion. *Food Chem.* 2007,102, 865–874.

[32] Wootton-Beard, P.C., Moran A., Ryan, L. Stability of the total antioxidant capacity and total polyphenol content of commercially available vegetable juices before and after *in vitro* digestion measured by FRAP, DPPH, ABTS and Folin–Ciocalteu methods. *Food Res. Int.* 2011, 44, 217–224.

[33] Rekha, C. R., Vijayalakshmi, G. Biomolecules and nutritional quality of soymilk fermented with probiotic yeast and bacteria. *Appl. Biochem. Biotechnol.* 2008, 151, 452–463.

[34] Jamali, B., Bjornsdottir, I.,Nordfang, O., Hansen, S.H. Investigation of racemisation of the enantiomers of glitazone drug compounds at different pH using chiral HPLC and chiral CE. *J. Pharm. Biom. Anal.* 2008, 46, 82−87.

[35] Dinnella, C., Minichino, P., D'Andrea, A.M., Monteleone, E. Bioaccessibility and antioxidant activity of phenolic compounds from extra-virgin olive oils during *in vitro* digestion. *J. Agric. Food. Chem.* 2007, 55, 8423–8429.

[36] Frontela-Saseta,C., Ruben- López, N., González-Bermúdez,C.A., Peso-Echarri,P., Ros-Berruezo, G., Martínez-Graciá, C., Canali, R., Virgili, F. Evaluation of antioxidant activity and antiproliferative effect of fruit juices enriched with pycnogenol in colon carcinoma cells. The effect of *in vitro* gastrointestinal digestion. *Phytother. Res.* 2011, 25, 1870–1875.

In: Functional Foods
Editors: Aron Robinson and Dominick Emerson ISBN: 978-1-62417-435-3

Chapter 6

MARKET STRATEGIES TO MAXIMISE CONSUMER ACCEPTANCE OF FUNCTIONAL DAIRY-BASED FOODS AND BEVERAGES

A. J. Troy[1], J. Bleiel[1] and J. Bogue[2]
[1]Food for Health Ireland, University College Cork
[2]Department of Food Business and Development,
University College Cork, Ireland

1. INTRODUCTION

The food industry generally, and the dairy industry specifically, are for the most part low-margin and extremely competitive businesses. Recent dairy industry trends have centered on food safety, product differentiation through quality, rigorous cost containment, careful inventory management, innovation management, and channel complexity (including the growing influence of retailers on the supply chain). However, as the demand for commodity dairy decreases in Western Europe, demand for dairy that offers health benefits - functional dairy - has never been greater. Dairy products can have vastly different characteristics, ranging from beverage to powder, solid to viscous, canned, bagged and boxed. Ingredients found in these products have been associated with a wide variety of health benefits and have been incorporated into a number of non-dairy based food and beverages as a means of increasing overall nutritional profile of the product (Deloitte, 2005). Consumer's increasing interest for maintaining and/or improving their health by eating these specific food products has led to the development of many new functional dairy products (Bhat and Bhat, 2011). However, not all of these products are met with consumer acceptance and product failure rate remains high. As sales of commodity dairy products slow in Western Europe, strategies that maximise and increase consumer acceptance of functional dairy foods and dairy ingredients are necessary to ensure a sustainable competitive advantage and ensure growth.

2. THE GLOBAL DAIRY MARKET

The demand for dairy products is expected to increase to mirror the continued growth in the population over the coming years (Teagasc, 2011). However, the level of demand is expected to differ based on product category and geographical location. The percentage share of each sector within the global dairy market for year ended 2009 is evident in Table 1 and clearly illustrates liquid milk as the market leader in terms of percentage share. Geographically, the demand for milk has been fuelled by a developing market for dairy (Datamonitor, 2010). Although, a low global compound annual growth rate (CAGR) of 1.9% is expected for the period 2011-2014, the Asia Pacific region is predicted to have a more positive CAGR during the same period at 3.5%. Western Europe is predicted to have the lowest CAGR of 0.2% (Van der Schraelen, 2010).

Table 1. Global dairy market segmentation: percentage share value 2009

Dairy type	Percentage share value
Milk	35.2
Cheese	28.3
Yogurt and Fromage Frais	17.1
Spreadable fats	11.4
Cream	4.7
Chilled desserts	3.3

Adapted from Datamonitor, 2010.

The second-largest sector in the dairy industry was cheese which grew by 3.6% in 2010. This represented a year on year reduction in growth from 5.5% in 2009 and 14.1% in 2008. The yoghurts and chilled desserts sectors experienced the greatest level of growth in 2010, and increased by 6.2% in terms of value from 2009. Aggressive promotion by retailers and increased interest in healthy eating among consumers helped maintain growth in the yoghurt sector in 2010 (Keynote, 2011).

3. THE EUROPEAN DAIRY MARKET

The dairy sector is of great importance to the European Union (EU) for a variety of reasons. The most striking feature of the EU is that milk is produced in all Member States without exception (European Communities, 2006). Within the EU to date, dairy companies have primarily focused their innovation efforts on products and less on marketing, organisation and process. Product innovations are mostly conducted on varieties. However, innovations in new ingredients (functional foods) have also been important (Siró *et al.*, 2008). Euromonitor (2010) confirmed that cheese offered the best growth potential over the five year period from 2010-2015 to Eastern European countries due to unrealised demand potential (Table 2). Yogurt, similar to cheese, has been driven more by value sales, particularly among younger consumers with increased spending potential. Liquid milk has registered slow growth and this is expected to continue.

Table 2. Forecast CAGR for European Dairy 2010-2015

European Dairy Product Category	Forecast CAGR 2010 - 2015
Soy beverages	10%
Cheese	6%
Yogurt	6%
Milk	4%
Other dairy	3%
Sour milk drinks	2%
Flavoured milk drinks	2%

Adapted from: Datamonitor, 2010.

4. FUNCTIONAL FOODS

Functional foods as a product category are often referred to as nutraceuticals (Global Regulatory Services, 2012). It is a diverse sector which spans across all product types and categories. A globally accepted definition for functional foods has yet to be agreed. However, the Food Safety Authority of Ireland regard a functional food as, a generally consumed foodstuff that may provide added health benefits, following the addition/concentration of a beneficial ingredient, or the removal/substitution of an ineffective or harmful ingredient (Food Safety Authority, Ireland, 2007). Functional foods are not intended to just satisfy hunger and provide necessary nutrients but may be used to improve the general wellbeing of an individual, such as prebiotics or probiotics, or decrease the risk of certain non-communicable diseases, such as cholesterol or blood pressure reduction (Siró *et al.,* 2008; Menrad *et al.,* 2003). Many studies have established that overall acceptance and interest in functional foods differed between countries and that understanding the needs and wants of the potential target market(s) was key to product success (Verbecke *et al.,* 2009; Bech-Larsen and Grunert, 2003; Urala *et al.,* 2003). Although milk represents the second largest segment of the global dairy market in terms of value, in the western world it is more premium priced, added-value drinks with built-in health benefits that are driving growth in dairy products. For the most part, these dairy products can be classified as functional products. Ingredients naturally found in dairy have been the focus of a variety of studies since first being focused upon in Japan in the early 1980s for the potential health benefits they offer consumers. These dairy components such as bioactive peptides, probiotic bacteria, antioxidants, vitamins and specific proteins have been found in yogurt and other fermented dairy foods, milk, colostrum, cheese, whey protein concentrates/isolates and milk protein concentrates (Bhat and Bhat, 2011). This has led to dairy becoming the largest functional foods and drinks category by most estimates, representing approximately 40% of the global market and up to 70% of the market in the UK and Europe (Mintel, 2011).

4.1. The Functional Dairy Market

Probiotic and prebiotic yoghurt drinks are one of the most well-known functional beverage products on the market. Probiotics can be defined as live micro-organisms that confer a health benefit to the host when they are consumed (Ziemer and Gibson, 1998). They are preparations or products which contain single or multiple cultures of bacteria (Bansal and Garg, 2008). Many studies have explained probiotic therapy as the administration of live micro-organisms for health-maintenance and disease prevention or treatment (Bansal and Garg, 2008; Reid, 2000). Yakult Honsha was the first company to launch the first probiotic drinking yoghurt, manufactured using fermented milk containing live lactic-acid bacteria, in Japan in 1935. This was soon followed by other major players in the dairy industry such as Danone, with brands such as *Activia* and *Actimel*, and *Müller*. Functional milks, are also a growing sector within the beverage industry. These milk products are fortified with a variety of functional ingredients including plant stanols, omega fatty acids, calcium and vitamins. There has also been a growth in the development of low allergen dairy products such as lactose free milk and soya milk to cater for the growing segment of consumers that wish to avoid ingredients associated with allergies (Mintel, 2011).

4.2. Consumer Acceptance of Functional Foods

The functional food sector has experienced major growth around the world (Datamonitor, 2009; JD Ford, 2009) but, it remains a niche category. International Markets Bureau (2009) stressed how the functional food industry reflected a shift from a mass market to a market with differentiated products that served a number of groups of consumers. The increasing cost of healthcare, steady increase in life expectancy and increased desire for quality in older age has encouraged consumers to address their intake of certain foods and beverages. It has motivated manufacturers to invest in the NPD of novel functional foods and beverages that address the growing needs and concerns of the increasingly health conscious population. Dairy-based functional foods and foods enriched with dairy-based ingredients have been at the forefront of the functional food category.

4.3. Consumer Acceptance of Functional Dairy Products

Within Europe consumer perceptions towards dairy products varies considerably. Consumer attitudes regarding dairy and weight-gain (Nolan-Clarke, 2011), heart-health, visual appearance (MilwardBrown, 2011), energy, muscle health (Nielsen 2007) and bone health (Huth et al., 2005) have all been well documented. However, a number of these studies have found specific perceptions are associated with specific dairy products. Urala and Lahteenmaki (2007) concluded that the reason for this was because consumers tended not to view functional foods or health giving foods as a homogenous product category, rather each product was assessed individually.

Perceptions towards carriers for functional ingredients or base products have been found to influence consumers' acceptance levels of functional dairy products. Products that are perceived as intrinsically healthy are normally viewed as credible carriers of functional foods (Coman, 2012). This belief has positively affected the functional yogurt segment. From a strategic perspective consideration must also be taken to ensure that the base carrier and the enrichment ingredient fit well together (Halliday, 2010). When this consideration is not taken into account it increases the risk of product failure at market launch stage. For example, if a perceived unhealthy carrier such as chocolate is enriched with a healthy ingredient such as Vitamin C the consumer is provided with a mixed message which can result in confusion and ultimate rejection of the product. Within the dairy industry it has been found that the enrichment of omega-3 was found to generate positive attitudes in dairy spreads, but negative attitudes in yogurt (Kolanowski and Laufenberg, 2006).

Table 3. European innovation trends by product type

Product Type	European Innovation Trends
Liquid milk	Reduced fat Healthy cholesterol New flavours Organic
Cheese	Reduced portion sizes, Reduced fat, Specialised flavours, Convenience
Yogurts	Probiotic Immunity New flavours Convenience Shots
Butter	Healthy cholesterol Natural Organic

(Adapted from Mintel 2010; Innova Insights 2010, Hall, 2007).

4.4. NPD in Dairy Ingredients and Products

New product development within the dairy industry has primarily focused on the development of products that were reduced in fat content and capable of supporting a hard (scientifically substantiated) health claim. The ability to market a health claim on a product package offered international food and beverage firms the opportunity to increase their return on investment (Cavaliar-Smith, 2012). However, as it has become more difficult in the EU to adhere to guidelines put forward by the European Food Safety Authority (EFSA), food and beverage producers have begun to look at methods of increasing return on investment through other means and more passive or soft claims. Innova Market Insights reported a 4% decline in the number of active health launches (e,g, fortified and functional) in Western Europe in 2010. For the same period there was an increase of 25% recorded for passive claim launches (food minus). As the demand for functional foods is steered more towards natural and inherent healthiness, dairy products provide manufacturers with a significant marketing opportunity (Mintel, 2010). For example, consumers' current interpretation of the term 'natural' is almost on an equal par with healthy and for this reason is a very valuable marketing term for the dairy industry. The National Dairy Council (NDC, 2012) of Ireland found that 74-79% of consumers believed that dairy was a natural unprocessed food. Recent new product introductions have utilised this information and have focused on the inherent natural qualities of dairy in addition to simple clean packaging that reflects the concept of 'natural' (Innova Insights, 2011).

Recent NPD within Europe (see Table 3) has focused on the development of healthier milks that addressed issues such as lower fat and reduced cholesterol; organic milk with low fat varieties, single serve products and new flavourings (Hall, 2007). For cheese products, an orientation towards health and convenience has been evident. Interestingly, the strategic health positioning of cheese products has included not only lower fat alternatives but smaller portion controlled packages that enabled the consumption of regular fat cheese products but in more moderate portion sizes. Innovation within the yogurt sector was primarily through new flavours. Intense competition in differentiation of health benefits is evident in this category.

5. Focused Market Strategies for Dairy Based Functional Foods

Successful marketing strategies should increase consumer motivation to purchase a product and also identify a clear positioning of the product in the consumers' mind. Although research clearly indicates that consumers have a desire for foods and beverages that will increase the healthiness of their diet, product failure of foods with health benefits still remains high. Functional foods, particularly novel functional foods can be met with uncertainty from consumers with up to 70% of functional foods experiencing failure within the first 18 months of product launch (Aschemann-Witzel *et al.*, 2011; Byrne, 2011). New product failure can result from a poor marketing strategy where factors such as: poor segmentation of the market, failure to integrate the consumer into the NPD process, ill-conceived pricing strategies or muddled promotional campaigns can significantly impact upon consumers' willingness to purchase (Hsu, 2011).

Tailoring a marketing strategy to match the product type and the target market is a key consideration for dairy food and beverage firms. Although all products should be treated differently, general consumer perceptions may provide important insights about the overall dairy category and more specific product segments. Consumers' understanding and positive attitude towards the term 'natural' is something which can be incorporated on a general level for all dairy products. This term can be implied and mentioned on dairy products through the ingredients or the product packaging and can help tie dairy products, particularly those using a health positioning strategy, to fit within the health and wellness trend. On a more specific level, it is possible to segment the dairy market into three broad categories: commodity products, functional products and indulgent products (Figure 1). Each of these segments offers the consumer a set of clear product attributes that enables the consumer to interpret the value associated with purchasing the product and offers a clear marketing message. These attributes should be the cornerstone for developing the marketing strategy for specific dairy products. Commodity dairy products consist of low fat milks and own brand dairy products. The primary attribute associated with this category is reduced cost. As commodity products tend to be low involvement products, their primary means of differentiation is through price. Functional dairy products consist of dairy-based products that have a specific health benefit or non-dairy products with a dairy-based functional ingredient. Product examples include: cholesterol reducing yogurt drinks, gut health products, vitamin-enriched drinks and protein-enriched formulas. Attributes associated with this product category are: health, wellness, increased cost and convenience. Indulgent dairy products consist of dairy-based products that are primarily marketed on the basis of their sensory appeal. Product examples include: ice-cream, cream, full-fat butter, artisan cheeses and more recently certain Greek style yogurts. Attributes associated with this product category are sensory appeal and increased cost.

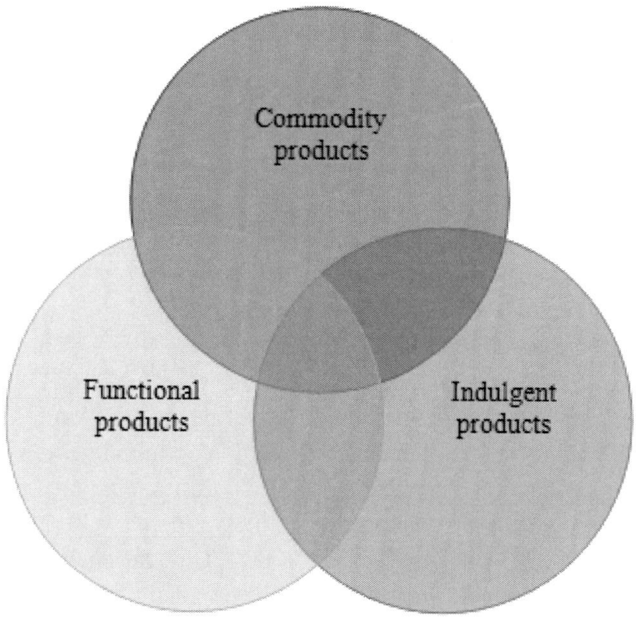

Figure 1. Segmentation of the dairy market .

However, a review of dairy products on the market would illustrate that a large number of products fail to clearly position themselves in one of these categories and instead find themselves situated in the overlap area between two clear cut segments (Nolan-Clarke, 2012; Yu, 2012). For example a commodity dairy product marketing health benefits for the heart or an ice-cream that has reduced fat content. These products are offering two messages to the consumer and, therefore, increase the likelihood that the consumer will become confused or will be unable to fully comprehend the value associated with the product in comparison to a competing product. It is important to understand the value chain in the consumers' mind with regard to dairy products. A wide variety of successful functional dairy products offer more than one benefit to the consumer. However, their marketing strategy clearly focuses on one particular benefit as the unique selling point. A current example is the *Chobani* Greek yogurt line. These products are clearly positioned within the indulgent dairy segment as the marketing strategy focuses on the taste and sensory appeal of the product. However, the product also offers a lower fat content than most other yogurts. This secondary benefit is not focused upon in the marketing campaign but rather the manufacturers use this secondary benefit to further convince the consumer about the value add of the product.

Conclusion

The global market clearly illustrates that the largest growth potential for milk is in developing markets (Datamonitor, 2010). The reduced consumption of liquid milk across developed markets has led producers to focus on the development of functional dairy products that appeal to consumers for their potential health benefits and links with overall wellness. The significant year on year growth in certain categories of dairy such as yogurt products and fermented dairy products in general corresponds to the health and wellness mega-trend which is dominating consumers' attitudes towards foods and beverages in developed countries (Euromonitor, 2010). Continued consumer acceptance of these functional products and novel functional products can only be achieved through a streamlined marketing strategy that offers a clear and consistent message to consumers.

Dairy based products that fall within the functional food segment and non-dairy based foods that are enriched with dairy ingredients should focus their marketing strategy on the primary benefit of health. Although a number of studies have found that the fat content of dairy is an important factor motivating product purchase, it becomes less important in the decision making process when another benefit, such as health, is marketed as the primary benefit. Such examples include: dairy-based yogurts with added plant stanols for cholesterol reduction. However, care should be taken to ensure that the health benefit is clearly understood by consumers. There has been evident where certain functional dairy products perform well in one market and poor in another. Ensuring that the benefit of the functional food is one which the target market can relate to and one which they desire is a method of ensuring demand for a product (Montague-Jones, 2011). Information provided on the package should also mirror the concept of health and wellness. Innova (2010) identified that the number of ingredients on a product label and the layout of the package contributed to the overall healthy image of a product. Products with clean and simple labels were perceived to be the healthiest by a large number of European consumers.

References

Aschemann-Witzel, J., Perez-Cuerto, F.J.A., Verbecke, W. and Bech-Larsen. T. (2011). Key success factors in health-related food marketing. A case study approach. Paper prepared for presentation at the EAAE 2011 Congress.

Bansal, T. and Garg, S. (2008). Probiotics: from functional foods to pharmaceutical probiotics. *Current Pharmaceutical Biotechnology,* Vol. 9, 4, p267 – 287.

Bech-Larsen, T. and Grunert, K.G. (2003). The perceived healthiness of functional foods – a conjoint study of Danish, Finnish and American consumers' perception of functional foods. *Appetite,* Vol. 40, p9-14.

Bhat, Z. and Bhat, H. (2011). Milk and dairy products as functional foods: A review. *International Journal of Dairy Science,* Vol. 6, p1-12.

Bowen, H.K., Clark, K.B., Holloway, C.A., and Wheelwright, S.C. (1994). Development projects: the engine of renewal. *Harvard Business Review,* Vol. 72, 5, p110-20.

Byrne, J. (2011). Heart health claims underscore functional cereal boom. Available from: http://www.bakeryandsnacks.com/Formulation/Heart-health-claims-underscore-functional-cereal-boom

Cavalier-Smith, N. (2012). Ingredients for success at Food Ingredients Europe, Paris. Paris: The Healthy Marketing Team.

Coman, M.M., Cecchini, C., Verdenelli, M.C., Silvi, S., Orpianesi, C. and Cresci, A. (2012). Functional foods as carriers for SYNBIO®, a probiotic bacteria combination. *International Journal of Food Microbiology,* Vol. 157, 3, p346-352.

Datamonitor. (2009). Tapping into the untapped drinks potential. London: IFIS Publishing.

Datamonitor. (2010). European Dairy. London: IFIS Publishing.

Datamonitor. (2010). Global Dairy. London: IFIS Publishing.

Deloitte. (2005). Profitable growth and value creation in the dairy industry: A view from Deloitte and SAP. Available from: http://www.deloitte.c om/assets/Dcom-Australia/Local%20Assets/Documents/White%20Paper_ Dairy(1).pdf.

Euromonitor. (2010). Strategies to exploit opportunities in global dairy. London: Euromonitor International.

European Communities. (1996). *Milk and milk products in the European Union.* Belguim: European Communities.

Food Safety Authority of Ireland (FSAI). (2007). Functional Food. Ireland: FSAI.Innova. (2010). *Fats and spread analysis.* Innova Market Insights.

Global Regulatory Services. (2012). Functional foods/nutraceuticals. Available from: http://www.globalregulatoryservices.com/industry-sectors/nutraceuticalsfunctional-foods.

Hall, R. (2007). Innovation and NPD in dairy. Business Insights.

Halliday. J. (2011). Arla and DMK for a new €44 million whey joint venture. Available from: http://www.nutraingredients.com/Industry/ Arla-and-DMK-form-new-44m-whey-joint-venture.

Hsu, Y. (2011). Design innovation and marketing strategies in successful product competition. *Emerald,* Vol. 26.

Innova Insights. (2010). *Fats and spread analysis.* Netherlands: Innova Market Insights

Innova Insights. (2011). *Worldwide trends in dairy.* Netherlands: Innova Market Insights.

International Markets Bureau. (2009). *Consumer trends, functional foods.* Canada: Agriculture and Agri-foods Canada.

JD Ford. (2009). *Global health and wellness: state of the industry.* Europe: JD Ford Marketing Company.

Keynote. (2011). *Milk and dairy products.* Teddington: Keynote Publications.

Kolanowski, W. and Laufenberg, G. (2006). Enrichment of food products with polyunsaturated fatty acids by fish oil addition. *European Food Research and Technology,* Vol. 222, 3-4, p471-477.

MilwardBrown. (2010). *Perceptions and insights on fats and fatty acids.* United States: MilwardBrown.

Mintel. (2010). *Butter, yellow fats and oils.* Mintel.

Mintel. (2011b). *Trends 2011 – dairy products.* Mintel.

Menrad, K. (2003). Market and marketing of functional food in Europe. *Journal of Food Engineering*, Vol. 56, 2-3, p181-188.

National Dairy Council. (2012). *Dairy for life.* Ireland: National Dairy Council.

Nielsen. (2007). *Organics and functional foods.* United States: Nielsen.

Nolan-Clark, D.J., Neale, E.P., Probst, Y.C., Charlton, K.E. and Tapsell, L.C. (2011). Consumers' salient beliefs regarding dairy products in the functional food era: A qualitative study using concepts from the theory of planned behaviour. *BMC Public Health,* Vol. 11, 843.

Safefood. (2008). *Consumer focused review – milk.* Ireland: Safefood.

Siró, I., Káplona, E., Káplona, B. and Lugasi, A. (2008). Functional food. Product development, marketing and consumer acceptance – a review. *Appetite,* Vol. 51, 3, p456-467.

Reid, G. (2000). Probiotic therapy and functional foods for prevention of urinary tract infections: state of the art science. *Current Infectious Disease,* Vol. 2, 6, p518-522.

Teagasc. (2011). News – Moorepark open day. Available from: http://www. teagasc.ie/news/2011/201106-02.asp.

Urala, N. (2008). *Why do consumers choose functional foods?* VTT Biotechnology, Consumer and Sensory Science. Available from: http://www.esn-network.com/657.html

Urala, N. and Lȧhteenmȧki, L. (2007). Consumers changing attitudes towards functional foods. *Food Quality and Preference*, Vol. 18, p1-12.

Van der Schraelen, T. (2010). What's hot and what's not in global dairy industry. Marketing Communication Manager, BENEO and Koen van Praet, Managing Director, Beneo Asia. Available from: http://www. timesinfomedia.com/cover_story/dairy.

Verbeke, W., Scholderer, J., and Lähteenmäki, L. (2009). Consumer appeal of nutrition and health claims in three existing product concepts. *Appetite,* Vol. 52, 3, p684-692.

Yu, D. (2010). Marketing Strategy for Small and Medium Sized Dairy Companies. *Value Engineering*, Vol. 29, 37.

Ziemer, C.J. and Gibson, G.R. (1998). An overview of probiotic, prebiotic and symbiotic in the functional food concept: perspectives and future strategies. *International Dairy Journal,* Vol. 8, 5, p473-479.

INDEX

A

B

C

D

H

I

J

K

L

P

Q

R

S

T

U

V